TRANSPLANTATION AND BLOOD TRANSFUSION

DEVELOPMENTS IN HEMATOLOGY AND IMMUNOLOGY

Lijnen, H.R., Collen, D. and Verstraete, M., eds: Synthetic Substrates in Clinical Blood Coagulation Assays. 1980. ISBN 90-247-2409-0

Smit Sibinga, C.Th., Das, P.C. and Forfar, J.O., eds: Paediatrics and Blood Transfusion. 1982. ISBN 90-247-2619-0

Fabris, N., ed: Immunology and Ageing. 1982. ISBN 90-247-2640-9

Hornstra, G.: Dietary Fats, Prostanoids and Arterial Thrombosis. 1982. ISBN 90-247-2667-0

Smit Sibinga, C.Th., Das, P.C. and Loghem, van J.J., eds: Blood Transfusion and Problems of Bleeding. 1982. ISBN 90-247-3058-9

Dormandy, J., ed: Red Cell Deformability and Filterability. 1983. ISBN 0-89838-578-4

Smit Sibinga, C.Th., Das, P.C. and Taswell, H.F., eds: Quality Assurance in Blood Banking and Its Clinical Impact. 1984. ISBN 0-89838-618-7

Besselaar, A.M.H.P. van den, Gralnick, H.R. and Lewis, S.M., eds: Thromboplastin Calibration and Oral Anticoagulant Control. 1984. ISBN 0-89838-637-3

Fondu, P. and Thijs, O., eds: Haemostatic Failure in Liver Disease. 1984. ISBN 0-89838-640-3

Smit Sibinga, C.Th., Das, P.C. and Opelz, G., eds: Transplantation and Blood Transfusion. 1984. ISBN 0-89838-686-1

Transplantation and Blood Transfusion

Proceedings of the Eighth Annual Symposium on Blood Transfusion, Groningen 1983, organized by the Red Cross Blood Bank Groningen-Drenthe

edited by

C.TH. SMIT SIBINGA and P.C. DAS

Red Cross Blood Bank Groningen-Drenthe
The Netherlands

G. OPELZ

Ruprecht Karls University
Heidelberg, FRG

1984 **MARTINUS NIJHOFF PUBLISHERS**
a member of the KLUWER ACADEMIC PUBLISHERS GROUP
BOSTON / DORDRECHT / LANCASTER

Distributors

for the United States and Canada: Kluwer Academic Publishers, 190 Old Derby Street, Hingham, MA 02043, USA
for the UK and Ireland: Kluwer Academic Publishers, MTP Press Limited, Falcon House, Queen Square, Lancaster LA1 1RN, England
for all other countries: Kluwer Academic Publishers Group, Distribution Center, P.O. Box 322, 3300 AH Dordrecht, The Netherlands

Library of Congress Cataloging in Publication Data

ISBN 0-89838-686-1 (this volume)
ISBN 90-247-2432-5 (series)

PRINTED IN THE NETHERLANDS

TRAVENOL

Acknowledgement

This publication has been made possible through the support of Travenol, which is gratefully acknowledged.

CONTENTS

INVITED SPEAKERS

D.W. van Bekkum (moderator)	- Radiological Institute TNO, Rijswijk, NL
W.L. Ford	- Dept. of Pathology, University of Manchester, UK
C.H. Gips	- Dept. of Internal Medicine, University of Groningen, Groningen, NL
A.B. Glassman (moderator)	- Medical University of South Carolina, Charleston SC, USA
J.M. Goldman	- Royal Postgraduate Medical School, University of London, London, UK
B. Griffith	- Dept. of Surgery, University of Pittsburgh, Pittsburgh PA, USA
G.F.J. Hendriks	- Universital Hospital Leiden, Leiden, NL
J.P. Hester	- University of Texas System Cancer Center, Houston TX, USA
W.G. Ho	- UCLA Hospital & Clinics, Los Angeles CA, USA
D.C.O. James	- The Anthony Nolan Bone Marrow Appeal, London, UK
G. Kootstra	- Dept. of General Surgery, University of Limburg, Maastricht, NL
M. Körbling (moderator)	- Ruprecht-Karls-University, Heidelberg, FRG
R.A.F. Krom	- Dept. of Surgery, University of Groningen, Groningen, NL
B. Löwenberg (moderator)	- Dr. Daniël den Hoed Cancer Centre, Rotterdam, NL
G. Opelz (chairman)	- Ruprecht-Karls-University, Heidelberg, FRG
G.G. Persijn	- Eurotransplant Foundation, University of Leiden, Leiden, NL
G.L. Phillips	- Barnard Cancer Center, Washington University, St. Louis MO, USA

R.J. Ploeg	- Dept. of Surgery, University of Leiden, Leiden, NL
K. Rolles	- Dept. of Surgery, University of Cambridge Clinical School, Cambridge, UK
R.T. Schooley	- Harvard Medical School, Massachusetts General Hospital, Boston MA, USA
H.G. de Vries-Hospers	- Laboratory for Medical Microbiology, University of Groningen, Groningen, NL
D. van der Waaij (moderator)	- Laboratory for Medical Microbiology, University of Groningen, Groningen, NL
J. van der Wijk (moderator)	- Dept. of Surgery, University of Groningen, Groningen, NL
R. Wood	- Nuffield Dept. of Surgery, University of Oxford, Oxford, UK

FOREWORD

G. Opelz

A comprehensive picture of organ transplantation is presented not only in terms of overall results, but also in terms of details concerning problem areas which are currently the subject of intensive research. Two very important aspects of organ transplantation have been emphasized. One is a multi-disciplinary thing, where collaboration and cooperation are essential. No single person or single group of people in any given department can do this. Organ transplantation needs a lot of supportive care and support from various disciplines. The Blood Banks play a particularly important role in this.

Secondly, transplantation has come of age. There is no question about it. The results that can be achieved today are so good that one can, without hesitation, say that transplantation has its place in today's clinical medicine. It is our job to convince the governments and granting agencies, the hospital administrators and the general public, that the money spent on these programmes is well spent. Although there is still room for improvement, there are many areas that can be identified where this programme has its clear function in medical treatment, today.

Much of the recent improvement has been attributed to cyclosporin A. There are some presentations with critical remarks to the effect that the usefulness of cyclosporin A has been overstated. I believe it is a good and important drug, but I would like to add two or three words of caution. I have sensed at various meetings, recently, a movement gaining momentum that I have termed "the cyclosporin in, immunology out movement", whereby some people seem to claim that if you use cyclosporin A you do not have to worry about anything anymore. To the contrary, from the preliminary data of the very large international kidney study that we are conducting – in which we now have data on over 8,000 patients that were transplanted in 1982 and 1983 – it looks like all immunological variables that one could identify with conventional treatment, also maintain their validity with cyclosporin A. That is, preformed antibodies, tissue typing, and most importantly the effect of blood transfusions. It has been claimed that with cyclosporin A, you do not need transfusions and you do not need to worry about them. The first results of patients treated with cyclosporin A show a huge difference between non-transfused and transfused patients. A comparison between non-transfused patients who either have received cyclosporin A or not, shows that the survival rate is exactly the same. In other words, cyclosporin A does not overcome the effect of transfusion. I think it is very important to stop this unfortunate development at an early stage. It is obviously important to try new things, but as one sees that the results end in disaster, it is better not to let this go too far.

OPENING ADDRESS

Prof.Dr. H. Vermey

As a representative of the Faculty of Medicine of the University of Groningen, it is a great honour and pleasure to be invited for an opening speech to this symposium, organized by the Red Cross Blood Bank Groningen-Drenthe.

This occasion symbolizes the exchange of ideas and cooperation which exist between the two institutions. It symbolizes too the relation between a University and a region.

With this eighth annual symposium, organized by the staff of the Blood Bank, a tradition is continued which originates from the ambition of this staff not only to offer a service in the field of patient care but also to fullfil a duty to inform users all over the region about new developments in the science of hemotherapy. In doing so this Blood Bank rises from a simple regional organization for supplying blood products to a higher level of functioning.

It takes the shape of an institute of applied science recognized as advanced medical care.

In the past years technical developments enabled us to produce a variety of blood components of high quality and high purity which provided a great efficiency to cope with growing demands for blood products. Many among us will remember the really primitive barracks on the University Hospital grounds, where this work was started. Still every year a symposium was organized.

This year, the topic will be Transplantation and Blood Transfusion, obviously not to misunderstand as a tautology since blood transfusion may be considered as a form of transplantation. A look at the programme shows you that after presentation of a number of basic principles more specific subjects will follow, making a comprehensive theme.

Today one may wonder if such expensive new developments in advanced medical technology and advanced patient care are justifiable and will survive in the present storm of shrinking expenditures.

Well, we all know that science is autonomous in its evolution and always new ways will open for further developments.

This holds equally for medical research. There has never been a way backwards, at most a delay; and delays have to be paid for.

The spin-off from new technology has unpredictably influence on the developments in many fields.

Even in a small country like The Netherlands participation in advanced medical research means preservation and support of basic scientific infrastructures. Here too the saying is, to make money you have to invest money.

Symposia like this one have the purpose to present the state of the art, but also to give an opportunity for discussion about the most important and relevant options. Therefore, I want to congratulate the organizing committee with the choice of this important theme and in bringing together in Groningen so many distinguished speakers and a great audience from all over the world.

I wish you a very good symposium with many fruitful discussions and many personal contacts.

I. PRINCIPLES IN TRANSPLANTATION PRACTICE

THE DEVELOPMENT OF THE LIVER TRANSPLANTATION TEAM IN GRONINGEN

C.H. Gips and R.A.F. Krom

INTRODUCTION

The liver transplant team in Groningen was in 1977 in an embryonic state. In 1978 the first patient was sent abroad to receive a new liver and in 1979 the first orthotopic liver transplantation was performed in an adult. More then three years later a child was transplanted a new liver. In 1983 the first patient from abroad came to receive a new liver in Groningen. By now, 31 orthotopic liver transplantations have been performed.

This article does not deal with skills and resources needed for liver transplantation. On this subject we have reported elsewhere (1). We here present some thoughts on features which we think have been pertinent to the development of our team.

OUTSET AND GOALS

Terminal liver disease is a matter of death. Liver transplantation is a matter of death and life. At the time we gathered thoughts about the start of our program, the one year survival rate was 20–35% in the major centres. Therefore, this treatment can only be undertaken by devoted personnel, who – in view of the high mortality – are able to carry on in realism and optimism. As the work is highly interdisciplinary (table I), the atmosphere in the hospital in and between departments has to be good. A potential major problem would be that in liver transplantation two types of donors are needed: organ donors and blood donors. Large amounts of blood products are used in some patients and when this would happen too often it might jeopardize both the Blood Bank and the transplant programme.

Table I. Team.

Multidisciplinary, involving:
academics, nurses, technicians
Secretaries of the following departments, institutes and laboratories:
anaesthesiology, blood bank, blood group serology, coagulation, clinical chemistry, clinical immunology, hematology, medical microbiology, medical pastorate, medical social work, nuclear medicine, pediatrics, pathology, radiology, revalidation, surgery, hepatology etc.

Although, because of the complicated procedure a "happy life forever" for all transplant patients without interference by the medical profession is not obtainable, high goals have to be set to improve quality. Our initial goal has been more modest – just to get our first patient alive and well from the operating table with a new liver. Even in this we did not succeed.

SPONSORING

Of major importance to our embryonic liver transplant team has been the sponsoring by two of the major centres, Denver (Thomas S. Starzl, now Pittsburgh) and Cambridge/London (Roy Y. Calne and Roger Williams). The two initial liver transplant surgeons in the team were trained in Denver and one of them is an experienced investigator in the field. Apart from transfer of surgical know-how, much anaesthesiological, medical, pathological-anatomical and immunological knowledge was obtained from these two (and other) centres.

Our zero patient received a new liver in 1978 in London. The team was there, participated in the follow-up and was supervised by the British team upon return of the patient to The Netherlands.

The support gave confidence to the team, hospital authorities and physicians who were to refer patients.

GROUP IDENTITY – INTERNAL COMMUNICATIONS

The liver transplant group had no specific personnel during the first four years of existance. Every member of the multidisciplinary team primarily had to do his own work and as an extra did her or his share in liver transplantation. At the same time this extra had to be done often at night, while no day of the week was excluded. The work is complicated and demands a great amount of self-discipline. As the group was small and loaded with enthousiasm, communication initially was easy. In a later phase meetings had to be held with the implicated disciplines. Apart from direct patient related problems, communication in the group is now effectuated by weekly liver transplant meetings, which are open to all group members and by a monthly newsletter. The hospital journal several times a year draws attention to events happening to the liver transplant group. The liver transplant group at the moment consists of about one hundred and twenty people, of whom 3.3 are paid as liver transplant employees. Group identity can only be achieved by generating and perpetuating enthousiasm in all people involved.

EVALUATION – MEDICAL AUDIT (MA)

On the weekly transplant meetings results are evaluated including bad results and team failures. The public, including the medical profession does regard liver transplantation as magic: the team and its patient are successful or not and there is little in between. Repealing this magic can only be achieved by the team because they are the only ones who know, even if their knowledge still is insufficient. Internal medicine audit therefore is of paramount importance and in the course of time this has improved the work of the team considerably. An example can be given. In some patients with cirrhosis of the liver the blood loss associated with the operation is so high, that this not only leads to increased mortality but is not justifiable for Blood Bank logistics, too.

Analysis of data showed that the patients with severe hepato-renal syndrome had the largest blood losses. It therefore was concluded that patients with cirrhosis of the liver should be operated before the development of severe hepato-renal syndrome.

Thereafter both the preoperative mortality and the amount of blood products used dropped substantially.

TEACHING

Liver transplantation has proved to be most attractive to medical students of our university. Several students have gone into projects related to liver transplantation as part of their teaching and the team has great benefit from these activities.

PROTOCOLLED MEDICAL PRACTICE

Protocolled medical practice is very important for any team. Initially, the protocols were diagnostic and open-ended, i.e. the diagnostic procedures were protocolled (blood and urine tests etc.), but not the frequency. In later protocols it also was stated on which days of which week tests etc. had to be performed. A standard therapy scheme (including immunosuppression) for the two weeks after transplantation was also included. The protocolled tests and the protocolled therapy do not have to be ordered separately and the results of the tests will appear automatically and independently to the department where the patient is hospitalized. The team does have more room to reflect and decide on the very complex problems which may come up after liver transplantation. For every cohort of ten patients a new protocol is made; the protocols provide in a five years follow-up. Protocolled is also the period immediately before transplantation. There is a specific preparative Blood Bank protocol providing in blood supply logistics (2).

PATIENTS AND RELATIVES

Patients who are terminally ill tend to accept a forty percent treatment mortality, where non-treatment results in 100% mortality. Therefore, they always will be grateful for a liver transplant. Relatives will be thankful because everything has been done, even when transplantation proofs unsuccessful. These facts imply that the team has to be extremely self-critical (see Medical Audit). On the other hand much moral support is to be obtained from both patients and relatives.

DONORS

As a rule the donor liver is obtained through Eurotransplant. The procedure will not be discussed here. For the liver transplant program it is of paramount importance that enough donor livers become available.

However, blood donors are as important. Lack of blood products definitely limitates the transplant programme. Blood donations are being done on a voluntary basis in The Netherlands and the liver transplant team several times has acknowledged in writing her gratefulness to the Regional Blood Donor Society. This Society has always had a positive and supportive attitude to the liver transplant project, even when in earlier days large amounts of blood products were used on a single patient.

AUTHORITIES – POLITICS

Authorities were involved in increasingly large circles. They were made enthousiastic and became involved to such an extent that they were not able to step back. They had to do their work in their own circle and they had to open up for the next larger circle. By-passing in principle did not occur, but if progress was held up, the burden was laid on the authorities in the largest circle reached. The sequence has been:

1. the chairman of the department, which had to deliver the greatest initial effort – anaesthesiology, internal medicine and surgery;
2. the hospital authorities;
3. the Ministry of Education;
4. the Ministry of Health;
5. the university.

Authorities are needed because they will or will not give priority to a project and because they will or will not provide the means to pursue. The main problem has been that although the importance of the project was acknowledged rapidly and gave prestige as well, also in terms of scientific spin-off, money was not provided. Group identity certainly was enforced by feeling that some patients were really helped albeit at the cost of tremendous efforts, while on the other hand the struggle for the funding was ongoing. The first financial signal came from the hospital board and the first political financial signal now is coming from the Ministry of Health. In both cases the team, having exhausted its financial resources, had to stop the liver transplants for some months, thereby making clear to everybody that action is needed. The Consensus Meeting in Washington in 1983, where liver transplantation was declared to be a treatment modality and a positive report on liver transplantation by the National Health Council which is advisory to the Dutch Minister of Health, have been very helpful in this respect. Without different forms of political pressure, liver transplantation would not have succeeded and the liver transplant team would have ended her life by the end of 1983.

COMMUNICATIONS TO THE EXTERIOR

The first scientific communication by the team on clinical liver transplantation was a review article followed by a case report of the zero patient, transplanted in London (3–4). Both articles were written in English and aimed primarily to be read by internists. Hereafter, reference of patients started to come. The medical profession was informed by the abstracts in the annual progress reports published by the Netherlands Association of the Liver. In the Nederlands Tijdschrift voor Geneeskunde (5–7) an extensive report was published on the results of the first 6 liver transplantations. Thereafter the number of referrals increased sharply.

As to the lay public the team decided that it should cooperate with news media, but on their request only. Two liver transplantations have been performed in Groningen before the first reports appeared in the press. The first transplantation was unsuccessful, the second successful. The late involvement of the news media provided the team the possibility to concentrate on the problems related to the treatment of the patient and to cooperate with the press. Since then the contact with press, radio and television has been balanced: more frequent when the team needed support and less frequent in the mean time. We still adhere to the principle of cooperating on request for the benefit of the team.

LIVER FOUNDATION

Part of the communication to the society has been done by the Dutch Liver Foundation which was founded (1981) in the period, when the team was developing too. The Dutch Liver Foundation has done much to increase the interest for liver disease by the general public and liver transplantation has been one of the stimuli they used.

CONCLUSION

The Dutch Liver Transplant Team is still developing. Much has been achieved and much has to be done. Launching a large and expensive project against the economic trend is a risky affair and endurance is needed. When a team continues to feel motivated much can be withstood. Motivation has come from devotion of team members, from support by patients and relatives, from support by the hospital, from support by the Blood Donor Society and the Blood Bank, from support in the news media and also from authorities who had to be pressed to the utmost to let their recognition of the project be followed by financial support.

REFERENCES

1. Krom RAF, Gips CH. Skills and resources in liver transplantation. Hepatology 1984, in press.
2. Smit Sibinga CTh, Achterhof L, Waltje J, Swieringa J, Das PC. Blood Bank logistics in liver transplantation. In: Gips CH, Krom RAF eds. Orthotopic liver transplantation. The Hague: Martinus Nijhoff Publ., 1984 in press.
3. Krom RAF, Gips CH. Liver transplantation today. Neth J Med 1978;21:97–100.
4. MacDougall BRD, Johnson PJ, Williams R, et al. Liver transplantation in a 27-year-old female with familial HBsAg-positive hepatocellular carcinoma. Neth J Med 1978;21:101–16.
5. Gips CH, Krom RAF, Groot EG de. Het lot van 30 patiënten voor wie in de jaren 1977 t.m. 1979 een levertransplantatie is overwogen, die bij 7 van hen ook is uitgevoerd. Ned T Geneesk 1981;125:868–75.

6. Gips CH, Krom RAF, Houthoff HJ, Schuur KH. Indicatiestelling en procedure bij het verwijzen van patiënten voor levertransplantatie. Ned T Geneesk 1981;125:875–8.
7. Krom RAF, Gips CH, Kootstra G, Newton D. Zes levertransplantaties te Groningen verricht. Ned T Geneesk 1981;125:878–85.

ASPECTS OF GRAFTING AND REJECTION WITH SPECIAL REFERENCE TO THE TRANSPLANTATION OF LYMPHOCYTES

W.L. Ford

INTRODUCTION

An allograft involves the transfer of one part of an organism to a genetically dissimilar individual of the same species. The term embraces three situations which are radically different in their physical and biological characteristics. First, a whole organ may be grafted with its blood supply intact by anastomosing its blood vessels to suitable blood vessels in the recipient. Examples are skin grafts placed on suitably prepared beds in the recipient and thymus grafts placed under the kidney capsule where they soon acquire a new blood supply. Third, dissociated cells may be grafted by injecting them directly into the bloodstream. Obviously this is most appropriate when the donor cells are normally present in the bloodstream or are able to leave the bloodstream easily to enter their natural environment as is the case with grafts of lymphocytes or bone marrow.

It has usually been assumed that the mechanisms underlying the rejection of all three forms of graft are basically similar when allowance is made for such factors as the time taken for the blood and lymph vessels of a skin graft to regenerate. In some examples of allografting, e.g. skin grafts, a cell mediated immune response is entirely responsible for rejection while in other cases, e.g. the transfusion of incompatible blood cells, an antibody response is mainly responsible. In kidney transplantation a cell mediated immune response is generally responsible for rejection but when transplants have been placed in patients who already have a high titre of anti-donor type antibodies rapid rejection with prominent vascular damage is evident.

The first part of this review article is concerned with two aspects of cell mediated immunity directed against organ and tissue allografts. These are first: what is the identity of the cell in the graft itself which is responsible for triggering the host response? Second: now that the existence of at least two subsets of T cells is well established, precisely which T cells are required for graft rejection? The second part of this review is focussed on the more specific question of how dissociated cells such as lymphocytes and bone marrow cells are recognized and eliminated after transfusion into allogeneic hosts. It has become apparent that such grafts can be destroyed by an unconventional mechanism which probably does not apply to organ or tissue grafts.

THE IMMUNOGENIC CELL IN ORGAN AND TISSUE GRAFTS

The notion that the stimulus to the host's immune system is delivered not by all the cells in an organ graft but by a minority of specialized cells has been current for several decades especially in the form of the passenger leucocyte theory. In some organs and tissues a radiosensitive cell that had recently arrived from the blood appeared to be critically important in eliciting the rejection response (1,2).

The overriding importance of the HLA-D antigens in graft rejection and their limited distribution to B lymphocytes, activated macrophages, dendritic cells and a few other cell types indicates that most of the cells in an organ graft probably play little or no part in initiating the rejection process. Recently a great deal of work has been concerned with Ia positive, e.g. HLA-DR positive, dendritic cells which are found in a number of sites and for this reason are referred to by a number of aliases. These include the dendritic cells of the spleen (not the follicular dendritic cells which are Ia negative) (3); the interdigating cells in lymph nodes (4); veiled cells in lymph (5); Langerhans cells in the epidermis and similar Ia positive dendritic cells in the connective tissue of many organs (6). These cells are all believed to be recently derived from bone marrow procursors although the precise details of their life history are uncertain.

The current notion that this Ia positive dendritic cell may have a paramount role in the immunogenicity of grafts has been advanced first by the finding that in one way mixed lymphocyte cultures this cell is many times more potent in stimulating allogeneic lymphocytes than are other Ia positive cells such as B lymphocytes and some macrophages (7). Second the characteristics of the dendritic cell as reported by a number of laboratories (3,7) distinguish it from the macrophages in a number of important respects (Table I). However it remains unclear to what extent the macrophage and the dendritic cell are really distinct cell lineages since no information is available on the potential of each cell type for conversion to the other. In certain circumstances dendritic cells can be observed to contain phago-

Table I. Contrasts and similarities between macrophages and Ia positive dendritic cells (interdigitating cells, veiled cells).

	Dendritic Cell*	Macrophage
Phagocytosis *in vitro*	No	Yes
Ia expression (HLA-DR)	Abundant, constitutive	Often negative, inducible
C3 receptor, Fc receptor	No	Yes
Stimulation in mixed lymphocyte reaction	Extremely potent	Weak or absent
Accessory cell for oxidative mitogenesis	Yes	No
Accessory activity for other immune responses *in vitro*	Variable	Variable
Interleukin-1 production	Yes	Yes

* Many unrelated cells can assume a dendritic morphology. See text for definition.

cytosed material or to bind contact sensitisers to their cell surface but this cannot yet be reproduced in vitro. The idea that the dendritic cell is a subset of mononuclear phagocytic cells is still tenable.

If Ia positive dendritic cells in the graft are indeed primarily responsible for stimulating the hosts' immune system the question arises of how this could be exploited to prevent rejection. Langerhans cells may be particularly sensitive to U-V radiation (8) but because of the limited penetration of U-V radiation in tissue this would seem to be an impracticable approach in the case of kidney or heart allografts. Other possibilities include the application of anti-HLA-D monoclonal antibodies; monoclonal antibodies directed against other determinants specific to the dendritic cell and possibly culture conditions that are selectively unfavourable to the dendritic cell (9).

SUBSETS OF T CELLS RESPONSIBLE FOR GRAFT REJECTION

Lymphocytes taken from animals that have rejected an allograft are specifically cytotoxic in vitro for target cells bearing the same antigens as the graft (10). This was regarded as a great advance in transplantation immunology when it was discovered more than twenty years ago and it led to much detailed analysis of the mechanism of T cell cytotoxicity. However recent findings have suggested that this large body of work may be irrelevant to graft rejection because in rats or mice lacking T cells the ability to reject grafts can be restored by transfer of the helper T cell subset alone; the minority subset of T cells which includes the precursors of cytotoxic cells (OKT8 positive in man) is apparently not required for graft rejection, nor is there evidence that it acts synergistically with the majority subset (OKT4) in this particular respect (11,12).

Presumably the destructive phase of rejection requires the secretion of lymphokines after T helper cells have divided and differentiated to produce "sensitized" T cells. Whether other cell types including macrophages and perhaps rather indiscriminate natural killer cells are recruited to play an active part in graft destruction is still uncertain despite a lot of investigative effort. The function of cytotoxic T cells is now believed to be the elimination of the body's own infected cells.

A recently developed monoclonal antibody directed against rat lymphocytes (OX22) has split the helper T cell population into positive and negative fractions. Reactivity against a particular transplantation antigen is found in the positive subset but helper activity for B cells is present in the negative subset (13). This might be taken to mean that different sets of T cells respond to alloantigens or to non-transplantation antigens but on the other hand some T cell clones appear to have dual specificity for both a transplantation antigen and a conventional antigen (14). A likely possibility is that different helper T cells collaborate with cytotoxic T cell precursors and with B cells respectively. Satisfying as this may be, an explanation is still needed for the peculiar nature of T cell responses against the antigens of the major histocompatibility complex (15) and especially the high frequency of responders in non-immune animals (16).

THE REJECTION OF LYMPHOCYTES TRANSFERRED TO ALLOGENEIC RECIPIENTS

Since lymphocytes recirculate continuously from blood to lymph, transfered lymphocytes present a moving target to the immune system of the host. Their rejection or survival is usually measured by labelling them in vitro with a radioactive isotope such as ^{51}Cr-sodium chromate. When rejection occurs a deficit of the radioactivity associated with allogeneic cells is observed in the host's lymphatic tissues while in the kidneys, the plasma and the urine there is a surplus of radioactivity released from dying cells. Several groups are studying lymphocyte rejection in this way (17–19). A recent volume (1983:73) of Immunological Reviews was devoted to this subject.

After the injection of allogeneic lymphocytes an antibody response directed against transplantation antigens is generally found. Although the alloantibody response is thymus dependent (20) even athymic nude rats can produce a response to allogeneic T cells through a mechanism aptly called "suicidal collaboration" (21). The donor T cells apparently activate the host B cells as may be general in graft-versus-host reactions (22). However several characteristics of allogeneic lymphocyte cytotoxicity (ALC) by non-immunized rats or mice suggest that the alloantibody response is not always the mechanism of rejection:

1) The rejection of allogeneic cells begins very quickly after injection. Two groups have published that it begins within 3 hours and 6 hours respectively (23,24). Recently we have found clear evidence that it begins within 90 minutes (unpublished).
2) Allogeneic lymphocytes are destroyed within the lymphatic tissues particular the spleen and lymph nodes. The evidence for this comes partly from autoradiographic study of the host tissues in which donor cells are being destroyed. In rats the destruction is consistently much faster in the cervical lymph nodes than in the mesenteric lymph nodes (19,24). Lymphocytes are not destroyed in the bloodstream or in the liver.
3) Young rats at the normal age of weaning (21–22 days) display very weak ALC but the capacity develops quickly between 4 and 6 weeks of life to adult levels (18). By contrast the ability to produce an antibody response begins within a few days of birth.
4) After irradiation of the recipient ALC is only slightly impaired compared to the depression of antibody formation although more severe inhibition of ALC was found in mice at 2 weeks after irradiation.

If a specific alloantibody response is not necessary for ALC the most likely possibility is that cell-mediated immunity is responsible. However nude rats, which are completely deficient in their ability to reject skin allografts (25), are actually superior to euthymic rats in their ability to reject allogeneic lymphocytes rapidly (24). The possibility that donor T lymphocytes might play some active role in their own rejection was excluded by the findings that either specifically unresponsive T lymphocytes or indeed a purified population of B lymphocytes are readily rejected (20). What is more the vigour of allogeneic lymphocyte rejection is not positively related to the strength of cell mediated responses as assessed by mixed lymphocyte reactions or graft-versus-graft activity (18).

The mechanism responsible for the rapid rejection of lymphocytes by non-immunized recipients has recently been argued in terms of "natural" antibody elicited by cross-reacting antigens, like the natural isohemagglutinin against

ABO antigens or alternatively a "natural killer" mechanism, that is a non-adaptive mechanism of cellular recognition independent of immunoglobulin (19). In order to distinguish these possibilities we produced rats that were profoundly deficient in T cells, B cells and all immunoglobulins. This was achieved by treating nude rats from birth with a rabbit anti-μ chain serum in order to abort te development of their B cell system (26). To my personal surprise these rats were if anything even more effective than control nude rats in recognizing and destroying allogeneic lymphocytes (24). It is highly paradoxical that although lymphocytes are an absolute requirement for allograft rejection either by antibody or by cell mediated immunity yet in a situation where the graft consists of lymphocytes no host lymphocytes are required for rejection. In fact the fewer lymphocytes present in the host the faster is graft rejection (27).

This mechanism of ALC may fall outside the definition of specific acquired immunity since there is no evidence of any memory effect on second exposure. The same mechanism probably applies to allografts consisting of other dissociated cells such as bone marrow grafts since Cudkowicz and Bennett showed that most of the rules of ALC as listed here also apply to marrow grafts into irradiated allogeneic mice (28). Recently this form of cytotoxicity against bone marrow cells has been demonstrated in vitro as well as in vivo (29).

Although ALC falls into the general category of natural killer cell activity, that is non-adaptive destruction implemented by cellular contact, it is not necessarily closely related to NK activity as studied against tumour target cells. In the anti-μ serum treated nude rat the host cells responsible for the recognition of the donor lymphocytes could be macrophages, interdigitating/dendritic cells, pre T cells or NK cells if in fact the last exist as a separate lineage. Recent evidence tends to incriminate the interdigitating cell as the culprit since RNA and nuclear debris from the allogeneic lymphocytes are found in large amounts in these cells within the host's spleen and cervical lymph nodes (Fossum & Rolstad, unpublished). However more direct evidence will be required before this surprising idea can be accepted and its relevance to clinical transplantation of leucocytes and bone marrow is even more enigmatic.

In conclusion there is not a single set of "rules of rejection" for every form of transplantation since allogeneic cells, tissues or organs can be destroyed by antibody, by cell mediated immunity or by non-adaptive cellular cytotoxicity.

REFERENCES

1. Elkins WL. The interaction of donor and host lymphoid cells in the pathogenesis of renal cortical destruction induced by a "local" graft-versus-host reaction. J Exp Med 1966;123:103–18.
2. Lafferty KJ, Jones MAS. Reactions of the graft-versus-host type. Aust J Exp Biol Med Sci 1969;47:17.
3. Steinman RM, Witmer MD, Nussensweig MC, Gutchinov B, Austyn JM. Studies with a monoclonal antibody to mouse dendritic cells. Transplant Proc 1981;15:299–310.
4. Fossum S, Smith ME, Bell EB, Ford WL. The Architecture of Rat Lymph Nodes. III. The Lymph Nodes and lymph-borne cells of the congenitally athymic nude rat (rnu). Scand J Immunol 1980;12:421–32.

5. Pugh CW, Macpherson GG, Steer HW. Characterization of non-lymphoid cells derived from rat peripheral lymph. J Exp Med 1983;157:1758–79.
6. Fabre JW, Hart DNJ. Demonstration and characterization of Ia-positive dendritic cells in the interstitial connective tissues of rat heart and other tissues but not brain. J Exp Med 1981;154:347–61.
7. Mason DW, Pugh CW, Webb M. The rat mixed lymphocyte reaction: roles of a dendritic cell in intestinal lymph and T cell subsets defined by monoclonal antibodies. Immunology 1981;44:75–87.
8. Friedmann PS. The immunobiology of Langerhans cells. Immunology Today 1981:124–7.
9. Lafferty KJ, Prowse SJ, Agostino M, Simeonovic CJ. Modulation of tissue immunogenicity. Transplant Proc 1983;15:1366–70.
10. Rosenau W, Moon HD. Lysis of homologous cells by sensitized lymphocytes in tissue culture. J Natl Canc Inst 1981;27:471–83.
11. Loveland BE, Hogarth PM, Ceredig Rh, McKenzie IFC. Cells mediating graft reaction in the mouse. I. Lyt-1 cell, mediate skin graft reaction. J Exp Med 1981;153:1044–57.
12. Dallman MJ, Mason DW, Webb M. The roles of host and donor cells in the rejection of skin allografts by T cell-deprived rats injected with syngeneic T cells. Eur J Immunol 1982;12:511–8.
13. Spcikett GP, Brandon MR, Mason DW, Williams AF, Woollett GR. MRC-OX22, a monoclonal antibody that labels a new subset of T lymphocytes and reacts with the high nuclear molecular weight form of the leukocyte-common antigen. J Exp Med 1983;158:795–810.
14. Ben-Nun A, Lando Z, Dorf ME, Burakoff SJ. Analysis of cross-reactive antigen specific T cell clones. Specific recognition of two major histocompability complex (MHC) and two non-MHC antigens by a single clone. J Exp Med 1983;157:2147–53.
15. Miller JFAP, Vadas MA. The major histocompability complex: Influence on immune reactivity and T-lymphocyte activation. Scand J Immunol 1977;6: 771–8.
16. Ford WL, Simmonds SJ, Atkins RC. Early cellular events in a systemic graft-versus-host reaction. II. Autoradiographic estimates of the frequency of donor lymphocytes which respond to each Ag-B-determined antigen complex. J Exp Med 1975; 141:681–96.
17. Bainbridge DR. Elimination of allogeneic lymphocytes by mice. Imm Rev 1983;73:5–34.
18. Heslop BF, McNeilage J. Natural cytotoxicity: Early killing of allogeneic lymphocytes in rats. Imm Rev 1983;73:35–53.
19. Rolstad B, Ford WL. The rapid elimination of allogeneic lymphocytes: relationship to established mechanisms of immunity and to lymphocyte traffic. Imm Rev 1983;73:87–114.
20. Rolstad B, Ford WL. The alloantibody response to a strong transplantation antigen (Ag-B). Quantitative aspects and thymus dependence of the response. Transplantation 1974;17:416–23.
21. Piquet PF, Vassalli P. Fate of T Lymphocytes injected into immunodeficient allogeneic nude or semi-allogeneic nude or semi-allogeneic F_1 mice: correlation with manifestations of a graft-versus-host reaction. Imm Rev 1983;73:71–86.
22. Ford WL, Rolstad B, Fossum S, Hunt SV, Smith ME, Sparshott SM. The stimulus to host cell proliferation in graft-versus-host reactions. Scand J Immunol 1981;14:705–13.
23. McNeilage LJ, Heslop BF. Lymphocyte homing in syngeneic and insensi-

tized MHC compatible allogeneic hosts. 1. Evidence for both syngeneic self-recognition and early killing of allogeneic cells. Cell Immunol 1980;50:58–70.

24. Tonnesen B, Rolstad B. In vivo elimination of allogeneic lymphocytes in normal and T cell deficient rats. Elimination does not require T cells. Scand J Immunol 1983;17:303–12.
25. Festing MFW. Athymic nude rats (Rattus norvegicus). In: Gershwin ME, Merchant B, eds. Immunologic Defects in Laboratory Animals. Plenum Press 1981:267–81.
26. Bazin H, Platteau B, Beckers A, Pauwels R. Differential effect of neonatal injections of anti-μ or anti-antibodies on the synthesis of IgM, IgD, IgE, IgA, IgG_1, IgG_{2a}, IgG_{2b} and IgG_{2c} immunoglobulin classes. J Immunol 1978;21:2083–7.
27. Rolstad B, Bazin H, Kimber I, Marshall J, Sparshott SM, Ford WL. The rapid rejection of allogeneic lymphocytes by a non-adaptive cell mediated mechanism. MS to be published.
28. Cudkowicz G, Bennet, M. Peculiar immunobiology of bone marrow allografts. 1. Graft rejection by irradiated responder mice. J Exp Med 1971;134:83–102.
29. Rolstad B, Benestad H. The "natural resistance" to bone marrow allografts in rats. Demonstration of rapid in vivo clearance of and in vitro cytotoxic reaction to allogeneic bone marrow in non-immune normal and athymic nude rats. MS to be published.

THE DRw6 PHENOMENON IN RENAL TRANSPLANTATION*

G.F.J. Hendriks

INTRODUCTION

During the first 10 years, the selection of potential recipients of cadaveric renal grafts in Eurotransplant was based primarily on ABO-compatibility and matching for the HLA-A and HLA-B locus determinants (1). The beneficial effect of HLA-A and -B matching on kidney graft survival was strongest in male recipients lacking bloodgroup O (2). HLA-A and -B matching did not only improve long term graft survival but also patient survival (3), probably due to a lower amount of corticosteroids given during the first postoperative months (4). However, 5 years after transplantation, over 40% of poorly matched grafts (those with ≥ 2 A/B mismatches) are still functioning. These recipients seem to be low responders against foreign transplantation antigens present in the graft. Another explanation may be that these patients belong to the so-called corticosteroid-sensitive group in which renal graft prognosis is good (5). Nevertheless, one should avoid, if possible, a high number of HLA-A and -B mismatches because there is one report that recipients with long term survival of poorly matched grafts appear to be in a high risk group with respect to the evetual development of malignancies (6).

In 1978, at the end of the first decade of organ exchange in Eurotransplant, HLA-DR typing of donors and recipient was introduced. Subsequently, all patients on the waiting list were typed for the HLA-A, -B, and -DR determinants, and in addition these patients had to be transfused prior to transplantation (7). The beneficial effect of HLA-DR matching on graft survival has been shown in several but not all transplant studies (8–10). One of the reasons may be that HLA-DR typing, especially of cadaveric donors, is difficult (11). Although blood transfusions and HLA-A, B matching improved graft survival, nevertheless approximately one-third of all grafts are lost during the first year after transplantation, mainly due to graft rejection. Consequently, defining whether or not a potential recipient is a high responder against transplantation antigens should be one of our first priorities. The usual way of measuring the control of immune response is by determining the humoral response, c.q. the formation of antibodies. DRw6

* This work was in part supported by the Dutch Foundation for Medical Research (FUNGO) which is subsidized by the Dutch Organization for the Advancement of Pure Research (ZWO), the J.A. Cohen Institute for Radiopathology and Radiation Protection (IRS) and the Kuratorium für Heimdialyse Neu Isenburg, Germany.

positive individuals are high responders with respect to the formation of antibodies against Streptococcal-antigens, non-MHC-antigens, Rhesus-antigens, and antigens present on B cells and monocytes (DR antigens) (12–15). DRw6 positive recipients of first and second renal allografts showed a significantly worse graft survival compared to recipients lacking the DRw6-gene (16). Some groups confirmed our findings, others did not (11, 17–19). The data mentioned above clearly show that DRw6 positive recipients are high responders after renal transplantation. As expected, matching for the HLA-DR determinants dramatically improved their graft survival (20). The excellent outcome of HLA-DR identical grafts, in DRw6 positive recipients prompted us to investigate the effect of the presence or absence of DRw6 in the organ donor on graft survival.

PATIENTS AND METHODS

The patients analysed in this study were transplanted between January 1978 and January 1982 within Eurotransplant. All patients received blood transfusions before transplantation. Only the recipients of primary renal allografts were selected for analysis. Patient death was considered as graft failure. Non-immunological failures were not excluded. For the analyses of the effect of the presence or absence of DRw6 in the donor on graft survival, only donors with two clearly defined HLA-DR specificities were selected. Most of the donors were retyped in the National Reference Centre in Leiden. Donors and recipients were typed with the standard Eurotransplant serum set for the HLA-A, -B, and -DR antigens. The HLA-A, -B typings were carried out with the standard NIH lymphocytotoxicity test (21) and the DR typings with the two colour fluorescence method (22). The serological definition of DRw6 was based on positive reactions with LB-E12 (MB1), MT2, and DR2+w6 antisera (23). This definition was consistent throughout the period in which the donors and recipients were typed. Graft survival times were calculated by the actuarial life-table method. The significance of the differences between groups of patients were tested with a chi-square derived from a long-rank analysis (24).

RESULTS

The overall beneficial effect of DR-matching in the total group of 1792 recipients is shown in table I. A difference of 13% in graft survival at one year between the DR-identical and 2 DR mismatched grafts was observed,

Table I. Actuarial life table estimates of probability (%) of graft survival.

Number of DR mismatches	Graft survival at 1 year
0	77
1	69
2	64
N=1792	p=0.00003

which is highly significant (p=0.00003). However, a completely different effect of DR-matching on graft survival is observed when the total group is subdivided with respect to the presence or absence of DRw6 in the donors and recipients. A highly significant beneficial effect of DR-matching is observed only in the group of 422 DRw6 positive recipients (table II).

Table II. Actuarial life table estimates of probability (%) of graft survival at 1 year in 422 DRw6 positive recipients.

Number of DR mismatch	Donor DRw6 positive	Donor DRw6 negative	All donors
0	82		82
1	80	59	68
2		51	51
	N.S.	N.S.	p=0.0003

The 1 year survival in the group of DR-identical grafts (DRw6 positive donors) is 82% versus 51% in the group with 2 DR mismatches (DRw6 negative donors). This difference is highly significant (p=0.0003). DRw6 positive recipients of 1 DR mismatched grafts showed a significantly better graft prognosis at 1 year if they had DRw6 positive rather than DRw6 negative donors (80% versus 59%, table II). Only a slight beneficial effect of DR mismatching in the total group of DRw6 negative recipients is observed (6% difference in graft survival at 1 year between the DR-identical and 1 DR, or 2 DR mismatched grafts (table III). In this group a similar pattern was found with respect to the presence or absence of DRw6 in the donor, namely, a better graft prognosis in the presence of 1 or 2 DR mismatches when the donors are DRw6 positive, than when they are DRw6 negative (table III).

Table III. Actuarial life table estimates of probability (%) of graft survival at 1 year in 1370 DRw6 negative recipients.

Number of DR mismatches	Donor DRw6 positive	Donor DRw6 negative	All donors
0		75	75
1	78	67	69
2	75	66	69
	N.S.	p=0.0006	p=0.007

DISCUSSION

It is a well established fact that grafts exchanged between HLA-identical donor recipient combinations require less immunosuppression and survive better than grafts obtained from cadaveric donors. Although servere rejection episodes can be treated successfully and graft survival may be sustained, every acute rejection episode leads to loss of functional nephrons. Moreover, severe side effects and complications due to excessive levels of corticosteroid therapy may occur. Recently, it was shown that DRw6 positive recipients are high responders after renal transplantation as illustrated by a higher incidence of irreversible rejections (15,17,19). Although these acute rejection episodes proved to be corticosteroid resistant, they were successfully reversed by treatment with rabbit-ATG (17). That fact clearly illustrates that transplant survival at 1 year is not always correlated with low responsiveness during the first post operative months. However, it is a possible explanation why certain centers were unable to confirm our findings, while other centers could do so. The suggestion that DRw6 may be a marker for an immune response gene has been criticized on the grounds that recognition why DRw6 is difficult, if not impossible. That is the reason why DRw6 had been excluded from certain transplant studies (9,10). However, sera have become available which makes the definition of this antigen quite reliable (23). The definition of DRw6 is based on positive reactions of MB1, MT2 and DR2+w6 antisera. The most important sera are the anti-MB1 sera which recognise an antigen coded for by the MB-locus which is closely linked to but separate from the DR-locus. MB1 is in strong linkage desequilibrium not only with DRw6, but also with DR1, DR2 and DRw10 in caucasoids (table IV). The phenotype frequency of DRw6 in random caucasoids is 25%. The DRw6-phenotype frequencies of the organ donors and recipients analysed in this study are 26% and 24% respectively.

Table IV. The relation between DR-MB-MT in caucasoid population.

	Associated DR-specificities
MB1 ≃ MT1 ≃ LB-E12 ≃ DC1	DR1, 2, w6, w10
MB2 ≃ LB-E17 ≃ DC3	DR3, 7
MB3 ≃ MT4 ≃ LB-E13 ≃ DC4	DR4, 5, w9
	Included DR-specificities
MT2	DR3, 5, w6, w8
MT3	DR4, 7, w9

As shown in table II, DR matching significantly improves graft survival only in DRw6 positive recipients. However, this strong beneficial effect is due to the presence of DRw6 in the donor which lead to excellent graft survival in the group of DR-identical and 1-DR mismatched donor/recipient pairs. The same "donor DRw6 phenomenon" is observed in DRw6 negative recipients of 1-DR and 2-DR mismatched grafts. It is very unlikely that the presence of a null gene leads to such a good graft survival in unrelated donor/recipient combinations. These facts logically lead to the question as to whether the "DRw6 donor phenomenon" is due to DRw6 or to MB1 which is used to define it. Data from intrafamilial kidney transplants suggest that the MB antigens strongly influence the survival of HLA-haplotype mismatched related grafts (25).

The overall better prognosis of DRw6 positive grafts can be explained only by assuming that the presence of DRw6 in the donor activates an unknown mechanism which suppresses the homograft reaction. This concept is not new. Low responsiveness to Streptococcal antigens is associated with MB1 and is suppressor T cell dependent (26). Other investigators showed that the induction of cytotoxic T cells could be inhibited by a monoclonal anti MB1 antibody (27). Antigens presented together with allogeneic class

II molecules (DR and MB determinants) stimulate predominantly T lymphocytes. The regulation of immune response occurs in two ways, through helper and suppressor effects. Therefore a low responder can be the result of either a lack of help or of active suppression. Antigens presented with DR may activate primarily the helper circuit, and those which are presented with some MB/MT antigens the suppressor/cytotoxic circuit. DRw6 may influence the homograft reaction in two very significant ways. Firstly, it may act as an immune response gene in recipients of renal allografts, and secondly by activating or inducing suppressor cell circuits. We cannot say whether either of the two processes is due to the DRw6 gene coded for by the DR-locus or the MB1 gene coded for by the MB-locus.

Our findings have important clinical implications. DRw6 positive recipients should be well matched for all DR antigens and especially for DRw6. A mismatch for DRw6, either alone or in combination with a mismatch for another DR-antigen confers an excellent prognosis for renal allografts in DRw6 negative recipients. Approximately 75% of all organ donors are DRw6 negative and should be preferentially transplanted in DRw6 negative recipients. Graft prognosis in this group of DRw6 negative donor/recipient pairs can substantially be improved by matching not only for the HLA-DR antigens but also for HLA-A and B antigens.

ACKNOWLEDGEMENTS

We could not have done this analysis without the generous support of the physicans collaborating in Eurotransplant. We thank the staff of the Department of Immunohaematology for technical help and Miss V. Diepeveen for preparing this manuscript.

REFERENCES

1. Rood JJ van. A proposal for international cooperation in organ transplantation. Histocompatibility Testing, 1967:451–2.
2. Opelz G, Terasaki PI. Influence of sex on histocompatibility matching in renal transplantation. Lancet 1977;i:419–21.
3. Persijn GG, Cohen B, Lansbergen Q, et al. Effect of HLA-A and HLA-B matching on survival of grafts and recipients after renal transplantation. N Engl J Med 1982;307:905–8.
4. Hooff JP van, Es JP van, Persijn GG, et al. Cadaveric graft survival, clinical course, blood transfusions, HLA (A and B) match, and DR match in adult patients transplanted in one center. Proceedings EDTA Congress, Robinson BHB, Hawkins JB, Naik RB, eds. Tunbridge Wells UK, Pitman Med Publ Co Ltd, 1979:359–65.
5. Dumble LJ, Clunie GJA, Macdonald M, Bowes G, Kincaid-Smith P. Prediction of renal allograft rejection response to steroids from ADCC response to in vitro steroids. Transplantation Proceedings 1983;15: 1145–7.
6. Birkeland SA. Malignant tumors in renal transplant patients; the scandia transplant material. Cancer 1983;51:1571–5.
7. Persijn GG. Immune modulation aspects of bloodtransfusion in transplantation practice. In: Smit Sibinga CTh, Das PC, Opelz G, eds. Transplantation and blood transfusion. The Hague: Martinus Nijhoff Publ. 1984: 43–56.

8. Persijn GG, Leeuwen A van, Hoogeboom J, Gabb BW, Nagtegaal A, Rood JJ van. Matching for HLA antigens of A, B, and DR loci in renal transplantation by Eurotransplant. Lancet 1978;ii:1278–81.
9. Berg B, Groth CG, Lundgren G, Möller E, Ringden O, Wilczek H. Five-year experience with DR matching in cadaveric kidney transplantation. Transplantation Proceedings 1983;15:1132–5.
10. Opelz G, Terasaki PI. International study of histocompatibility in renal transplantation. Transplantation 1982;33,1:87–95.
11. Jakobsen B, Langhoff E, Platz P, et al. The impact of HLA-DR compatibility on cadaver kidney graft survival in a prospective study with special emphasis on the quality of typing. Tissue Antigens 1984;23:94–104.
12. Lehner T. The relationship between human helper and suppressor factors to a streptococcal protein antigen. J Immunology 1982;129:1936–40.
13. Baldwin WM, Claas FHJ, Es LA van, Rood JJ van, Paul LC, Persijn GG. Renal graft rejection and the antigenic anatomy of human kidneys. Proceedings of the thirteenth International Course on Transplantation and Clinical Immunology, Lyon 1981;13:140–6.
14. Darke C, Street J, Sargeant C, Dyer PA. HLA-DR antigens and properdin factor B allotypes in responders and non-responders to the Rhesus-D antigen. Tissue Antigens 1983;21:333–5.
15. Hendriks GFJ, Claas FHJ, Persijn GG, Witvliet MD, Baldwin W, Rood JJ van. HLA-DRw6 positive recipients are high responders in renal transplantation. Transplantation Proceedings 1983;15:1136–8.
16. Hendriks GFJ, Scheuder GMTh, Claas FHJ, et al. HLA-DRw6 and renal allograft rejection. Brit Med J 1983;286:85–7.
17. Hoitsma HJ, Reekers P, Lier HJJ van, Rens JG van, Koene R. HLA-Drw6 and treatment of acute rejection with antithymocyte globulin in renal transplantation. Transplantation 1984, in press.
18. Soulilou JP, Bignon JD. Poor kidney graft survival in recipients with HLA-DRw6. N Engl J Ned 1983;308:969.
19. Schmidt P, Balcke P, Zazgornik J, et al. HLA-DRw6 matching and primary renal graft failure due to rejection. Lancet 1983;ii:1277
20. Hendriks GFJ, Claas FHJ, Schreuder GMTh, et al. Influence of HLA-DRw6 and HLA-DR matching on kidney graft prognosis. Dialysis & Transplantation 1983;12:95–6.
21. Ray JG. NIH lymphocyte microcytotoxicity technique. NIAID manual of tissue typing techniques (DHEW publication no (NIH) 77-545) DHEW 1977:32.
22. Rood JJ van, Leeuwen A van, Ploem JS. Simultaneous detection of two cell populations by two-colour fluorescence and application to the recognition of B-cell determinants. Nature 1976;262:795–7.
23. Schreuder GMTh, Parlevliet J, Termijtelen A, Rood JJ van. Reanalysis of the HLA-DRw6 complex. Tissue Antigens 1983;21:62–74.
24. Peto R, Pike MC, Armitage P, et al. Design and analysis of randomized clinical trials requiring prolonged observation of each patient. II. Analysis and examples. Brit J Cancer 1977;35:1–39.
25. Duquesnoy RJ, Annen KB, Marrari MM, Kauffman jr HM. Association of MB compatibility with successfull intrafamilial kidney transplantation. N Eng J Med 1980;302:821–4.
26. Nishimura Y, Sasazuki T. Suppressor T cells control the HLA linked low responsiveness to streptococcal antigen in man. Nature 1983;302:67–9.
27. Corte G, Moretta A, Cosulich ME, Ramarli D, Bargellese A. A monoclonal anti-DC1 antibody selectively inhibits the generation of effector T cells mediating specific cytolytic activity. J Exp Med 1982;156:1539–44.

CRYOPRESERVATION OF PLATELETS, BONE MARROW AND LYMPHOCYTES: APPLICATIONS FOR THE TRANSPLANT RECIPIENT

A.B. Glassman

INTRODUCTION AND PURPOSE

Patients awaiting transplantation have a variety of hematologic disorders. This study examines the abnormalities encoutered and the cryopreserved blood elements that are available for therapy. Anemia is the most common hematologic disease noted in the renal transplant patient. The renal transplant patient receives more benefits from red blood cells that are not cryopreserved (1). Definitive studies as to the role of frozen deglycerolized red blood cells versus packed red cells or other products in patients awaiting other organ transplants such as liver or bone marrow are ongoing. Cryopreservation of red blood cells and the clinical application of this product will not be addressed in this work.

Thrombocytopenia and granulocytopenia can be major problems in the patient awaiting bone marrow transplantation. These conditions may exist prior to transplantation because of the underlying disease process, due to therapy for the disease or a combination of factors. Often following transplantation there are indications for platelets and granulocytes because of therapy to decrease graft rejection (2–4). Providing the platelets and granulocytes places demands on the immunohematology service. Cryopreservation of platelets is a clinically useful entity which has been available for several years and is growing in popularity (5–7). Granulocytes cannot be cryopreserved in a practical way except in liquid storage for short periods. There is increasing interest for the use of cryopreserved stem cells and bone marrow. These may be used as autologous bone marrow or allogeneic grafts.

The purposes of this paper are twofold. The first is to examine the cryobiology associated with the frozen preservation of platelets, granulocytes, lymphocytes, stem cells and bone marrow. The second is to provide the present clinical indications and applications with some speculations about future use.

METHODS AND CRYOBIOLOGICAL CONSIDERATIONS

A. General. Cellular injury occurs by two general mechanisms during freezing. One of these is chemical injury which occurs because of the loss of liquid water. As ice forms, it decreases the amount of liquid water which acts as a solvent. Chemicals which otherwise are in solution in liquid water become more concentrated as freezing takes place. There is, however, a great deal of variability among living systems for surviving the loss of intracellular water. Freezing is a type of dehydration. Ice in biological systems may lead to denaturation of large molecules especially certain proteins and enzymes. Sulfhydryl groups seem to be especially sensitive to the loss of water during ice formation. During dehydration, disulfide bonds may form causing enzymes and other proteins to lose their normal shape and interact with each other.

A second general mechanism by which cellular injury occurs during freezing is mechanical. This is the result of alteration of membrane characteristics of the frozen cells. Recent evidence indicates that membrane vesicles can be dehydrated in the presence of trehalose without the phase transitions that are usually seen with severe dehydration (8). Association of carbohydrates with phosphate head groups of phospholipids may involve changes such that membranes can remain functional after rehydration and avoid the oxidative damages to the dry membranes which otherwise would occur.

For cells to survive cryopreservation, they must be protected from mechanical and chemical sources of injury. This can be done through controlling the cooling rate. Ice forms in the extracellular space outside the cell membrane when slow cooling occurs. More rapid cooling may result in simultaneous intra and extra cellular ice formation. Vapor pressure for liquid water that is inside a slowly cooled cell is greater than the vapor pressure of ice. This greater vapor pressure of the liquid intracellular water forces the water through the cell membrane and out of the cell during slow cooling. Slow cooling may be defined as a rate of temperature decline sufficiently slow so that ice crystals are confined extracellularly. The specific cooling rate is determined for each type of cell under consideration. Cells highly permeable to water, such as the red blood cell, can lose water very quickly and therefore may be cooled more rapidly than cells which are less permeable to water, such as granulocytes and platelets. The accompanying graph illustrates the concept of slow cooling rate (Figure 1). An important aspect of controlling mechanical injury is to thaw cells fairly rapidly. Rapid thawing tends to prevent recrystalization. Recrystalization is the physical phenomenon whereby ice crystals grow larger as the subzero temperature becomes warmer. Since crystal growth is time dependent, the goal is to thaw rapidly enough so that there is insufficient time for intracellular ice crystals to grow to damaging proportions. The principle of rapid thawing is probably independent of cell type.

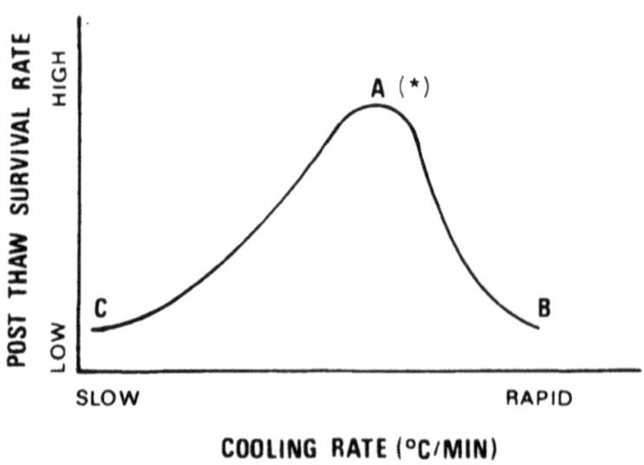

Figure 1. "Cooling rate vs. post thaw survival: hypothetical curve" Point A(*) indicates optimum cooling rate, maximal survival after thawing. (Redrawn from Glassman AB, Karow AM (9)).

B. Cryoprotectants: pharmacologic means of protecting cells during freezing. Physical factors of storage temperature, cooling and thawing rates are important to insure cell survival as already described. Cell survival can be further enhanced by the use of cryoprotectant agents. A cryoprotectant is by definition a substance which when applied to living cells before freezing yields a higher post thaw survival than could be obtained without that substance. There are two major classes of cryoprotectants: low molecular weight and high molecular weight. Dimethyl sulfoxide (DMSO) and glycerol are two important examples of low molecular weight cryoprotectants. Glycerol is the cryoprotectant used in red blood cell cryopreservation. DMSO has much greater importance for cryopreservation of platelets, lymphocytes, stem cells and bone marrow cells. High molecular weight cryoprotectants such as dextran, hydroxyethyl starch and polyvinylpyrrolidone are of interest in cryobiological research because lower concentrations of them are needed to achieve cryoprotection in certain kinds of cells.

The manner in which cryoprotectants act is obscure. It may involve a complex series of mechanisms which cause alteration of the freezing point, change in solute concentration, interaction of phospholipids within cellular and subcellular organelle membranes and alteration of cell volume preventing cell deformation and mechanical injury. It has been postulated that they may also act as direct surface coating agents protecting membranes which are particularly susceptible to freezing injury or by increasing the amount of nonfreezable liquid to prevent cellular shrinking and associated membrane stress. The entirety of the specific mechanisms of cryoprotectant action is not known. To be effective for cryopreservation, they must be in direct contact or within the cells. Cryoprotectants have the effect of decreasing optimum cooling rates as seen in the associated figure (Figure 2).

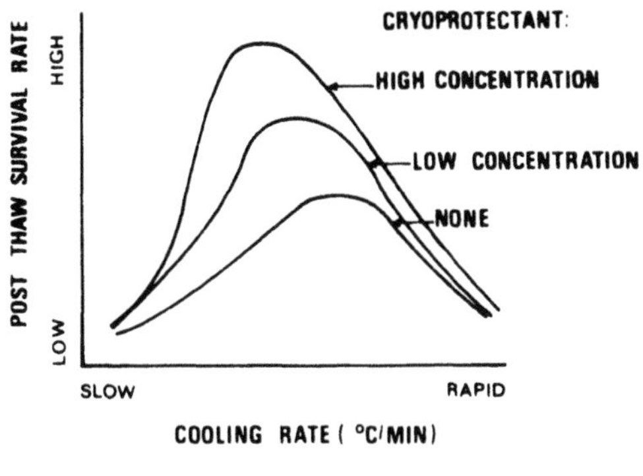

Figure 2. Varying concentrations of cryoprotectants on post thaw survival and cooling rate. (Redrawn from Glassman AB, Karow AM (9)).

The presence of a cryoprotectant results in an optimal cooling rate slower than the cooling rate without a cryoprotectant. The use of cryoprotectants makes the prevention of intracellular ice by the loss of water through slow cooling more likely. The proportion of cells surviving freezing is increased as the concentration of the cryoprotectant is increased to an optimum level.

Cryoprotectants can exert toxic effects when used in excess concentrations. These toxic effects at the extremely high concentrations reduce survival rate. Two other factors contribute to cryoprotectant toxicity: (1) warm temperatures (above 15°C) and; (2) duration of cellular exposure to the warm cryoprotectant.

THE USE OF CRYOPRESERVED BLOOD ELEMENTS IN THE TRANSPLANT PATIENT

A. Platelets

1. Indications. Thrombocytopenia is the indication for platelets. Platelet transfusions are given to correct hemostatic abnormalities in patients with inadequate numbers of effective platelets. Improperly functioning platelets associated with metabolic abnormalities such as chronic renal failure or severe liver disease will not be aided by the infusion of exogenous platelets. Indeed, the exogenous platelets may become metabolically impaired and will not result in any benefit for the patient. Thrombocytopenia must be treated effectively with the knowledge that the patient will have a proper increment both in quantity and in function of the transfused platelets. When thrombocytopenia is associated with specific platelet antibodies, the donor platelets must be antigenically compatible. Cryopreservation techniques can make platelets available for autologous transfusion. Where applicable, selection of HLA and/or platelet antigen compatible donor storage for later use could be arranged.

Thrombocytopenic patients with less than $20x10^9/l$ platelets usually have indications for platelet transfusion. Some patients may have platelet counts of less than $20x10^9/l$ platelets for periods of time without significant bleeding. Clinical hemorrhage is unusual with platelet counts of greater than $80x10^9/l$ platelets unless the platelets are functionally abnormal as when associated with severe metabolic disease states (renal and/or hepatic failure).

Platelets carry ABO antigens passively. Several studies have demonstrated that ABO incompatible platelets can provide hemostatic benefits to the patient. The compatibility of the donor plasma with recipient red cells which is a consideration in liquid platelets is not of concern for the cryopreserved platelets.

Patients receiving multiple platelet transfusion from random donors may become sensitized to platelet antigens. Cryopreserving platelets of specific antigenic compatibility is theoretically useful. The HLA as well as the platelet antigen systems appear to be significant in platelet transfusion (10–12). Freezing of autologous platelets has been recommended and may be useful particularly in selected bone marrow transplant patients.

2. Cryopreserved preparations. Platelets can be made available by cryopreservation in glycerol or DMSO. The most commonly used method is 5% DMSO preserved in liquid nitrogen. Post transfusion survival of cryopreserved and thawed platelets ranges from 40% to 50% or more. They appear to have good function and clinical utility (13–16).

Platelets do not remain viable for more than 120 hours in the liquid state at 22°C. Freezing of platelets with DMSO, glycerol, or hydroxyethyl starch seems to offer the greatest possibility for long-term storage of platelets for autologous use and random donor storage. Currently, the best method for cryopreserving platelets employs a slow cooling rate plus a 5% concentration of DMSO. This seems to offer the highest level of platelet recovery and survival (17).

3. Future use. Cryopreservation of platelets may be a method of providing autologous platelets for the bone marrow transplant patient of the future. The method using DMSO is clinically applicable and provides long term storage and greater availability of platelets to patients. There is emerging evidence that platelets are also active in a host defense mechanism role for bacteria and viruses. In the future there may be recommendations that bone marrow suppressed patients should be given a combination of platelets and granulocytes.

B. Stem cell and bone marrow

1. Indicatons. Clinical indications for bone marrow transplantation include bone marrow aplasia or hypoplasia in a spectrum of patients ranging from those with immunodeficiency diseases, aplastic anemia, leukemias through those who have been treated with chemo or radiation therapy. Bone marrow engraftment is expected to provide red cells and white cells replacing endogenous function (18). Significant cellular production from the graft is expected in approximately two weeks.

2. Cryopreserved preparations. Bone marrow and stem cells are well preserved either from autologous or allogeneic donors using approximately 10% dimethyl sulfoxide (DMSO). Data from studies done in our laboratory to evaluate effects of freezing on the proliferative response of cells in vitro confirms this. The methylcellulose clonal cell culture assay was used (19,20). Mouse and human bone marrow cells were placed in a freezing solution of 20% heat-inactivated fetal calf serum, 10% DMSO with 100 units per ml of penicillin-streptomycin in Alpha (α)-medium. The cell suspension was then placed in a programmable liquid nitrogen (LN_2) freezer and frozen at a cooling rate of 1°C per minute, with the liquid phase change occurring at -5°C. At the solid phase change, the freezing rate was 5°C per minute until -80°C. The samples were then transferred directly into liquid nitrogen (-196°C) cannisters until clonal cell culture assays were performed. The frozen cells were then thawed slowly, washed in tissue culture medium, counted, and then added to tissue culture assay (21,22). This method provided greater than 80% viability of bone marrow cells as determined by the in vitro method used to assay for colony forming units – granulocytes (CFU-C) and burst forming units – erythrocytes (BFU-E).

3. Clinical utility. Autologous bone marrow programmes are being set up in many medical centers at the present time (23–26). The advantage of this is that the patient can donate his/her bone marrow during a period of remission and then be treated very actively with chemo or radiation therapy. The patient receives autologous bone marrow without the risk of graft-versus-host reactions or rejection phenomenon. The use of autologous bone marrow may be indicated if the patient is able to donate early enough in the course of the disease, i.e. prior to bone marrow suppression or metastatic tumor involvement. Allogeneic bone marrow transplants require attention to HLA matching, mixed lymphocyte reactions and the problems of graft-versus-host complications.

Some patients may already have marrow metastases at time of autologous donation. Methods for early detection of metastases, tolerable numbers of cancer cells, if any, and differential ability of tumor cells to survive cryopreservation are being evaluated. The long range success of autologous bone marrow preservation and transportation will depend in part on the ability of the organ bank to answer these questions.

4. Future use. There will be expanded use of bone marrow and stem cell transplants in the future. HLA-identical, ABO-compatible and mixed lymphocyte culture unreactive donors will be chosen in those intances where autologous donations cannot be obtained. ABO matching in bone marrow transplants may not be as critical as for some other organs, particularly the kidney. At the present time, potential bone marrow recipients should not receive red blood cells or other blood components from potential donors or family members even if HLA identical because of the theoretical risk of sensitization to minor histocompatibility antigens. Graft rejection and graft versus host disease still ocur and are problems in bone marrow recipients. These reactions, at the present time, cause 10–20% fatility rate among human bone marrow recipients. Better tissue antigen matching including possible matching for sex chromosomes and eliminating of potential infectious agents (e.g. cytomegalic inclusion disease virus or CMV, herpes simplex virus, toxoplasmosis, etc.) may enhance future bone marrow transplant survival. Irradiation of blood products given to bone marrow recipients may reduce the incidence of graft-versus-host reactions (27).

C. Lymphocytes

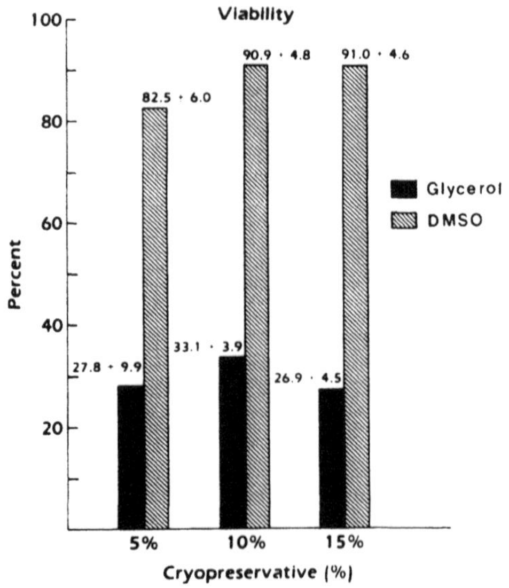

Figure 3. Lymphocyte viability relative to cryopreservative. (Drawn from data in Glassman AB, Bennett CE (26)).

1. Indications. Lymphocytes are used in mixed lymphocyte cultures to test HLA compatibility. Their use as reagent cells is expanding. Lymphocyte preparations are a source of dialyzable leukocyte extract and have been used in some protocols at our institution for the preparation of transfer factor.

2. Cryopreserved preparations. Lymphocytes survive LN_2 cryopreservation well in 10% DMSO. There is a greater than 85% post thawing viability as determined by trypan blue exclusion (Figure 3) (28).

Lymphocytes are isolated from whole blood by using the ficoll-hypaque gradient separation technique. The cells are then washed in medium, counted and assessed for viability by trypan blue exclusion. For freezing, cells are resuspended in 20% heat-inactivated fetal calf serum/RPMI 1640 to a minimum concentration of 5×10^6 cells/ml. Sterile, cold 100% DMSO is added very slowly to the cell suspension to a concentration of 10% with gentle mixing by Pasteur pipette; this allows the cryoprotectant (DMSO) to penetrate the cells. DMSO is toxic to most cell types at the concentration used for cryopreservation, therefore it is important to keep the cell suspension and the DMSO cold (4°C or on ice) before and after the addition of the cryoprotectant. This seems to reduce toxicity. Cells are placed in the programmable freezer and

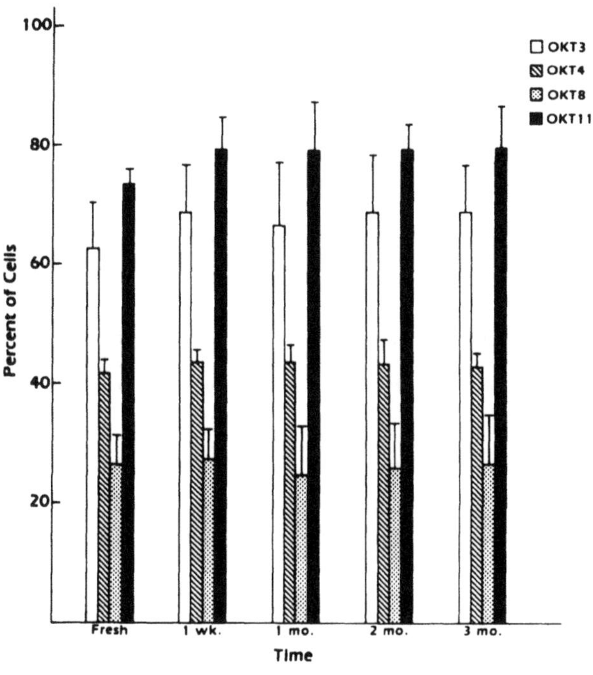

Figure 4. Comparison of fresh vs. cryopreserved T cell subpopulations measured by the ortho spectrum III.

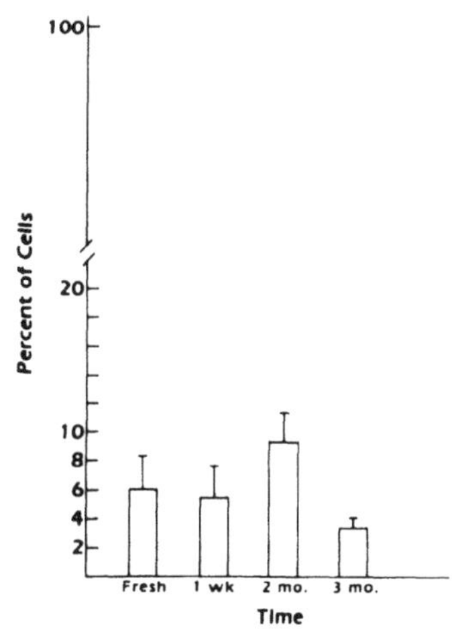

Figure 5. Comparison of fresh vs. cryopreserved B cells measured by the ortho spectrum III.

frozen at a slow cooling rate, usually 1°C per minute, then stored in liquid nitrogen (-196°C) (29). Freshly frozen lymphocytes retain their T subpopulations as measured by monoclonal antibodies, total B cells measured by a fluorescein conjugated polyvalent antiserum with B-cell specificity (Figures 4 and 5) and their lymphocyte blast transformation characteristics as measured by tritiated thymidine uptake (30,31).

3. Clinical utility. Clinical utility of cryopreserved lymphocytes is as reagent cells for antigen identification and use in mixed lymphocyte reactions. Infusion of lymphocytes into patients who are immunosuppressed may result in severe graft-versus-host reaction. There may be some stem cells obtained during the collection of lymphocytes with some of the mechanical collecting devices in use.

4. Future use. There will be an expanded demand for the use of lymphocytes as reagents, particularly in patients awaiting transplantation. Whether there will be continuing need for the use of lymphocyte preparations either as stem cells or for dialyzable leukocyte extract (transfer factor) remains speculative.

D. Granulocytes

1. Indications. The general indication for the clinical use of granulocytes is granulocytopenia of less than 0.25×10^9/l granulocytes in a patient who is refractory to antibiotic therapy which would otherwise be used to control bacterial infections and/or mycotic diseases.

2. Cryopreserved preparations. Because of the difficulties with the control of the intracellular osmotic pressure of the granulocyte, there are at the present time no practical methods of granulocyte cryopreservation. Granulocytes are available in a liquid form and probably have reasonable function for approximately 24 hours when kept at 4°C. Use of a variety of cryopreservative agents including glycerol and DMSO indicate no promising results for the future cryopreservation of human granulocytes (32).

3. Clinical utility. Cryopreservation of granulocytes is at present strictly a clinical investigative modality. There seems to be little or no demonstration of adequate fucntional human granulocytes after cryopreservation regardless of freezing rate, use of cryopreservative, temperature, storage or thawing.

4. Future use. The future support of the infected immunocompromised granulocytopenic patient who is about to undergo bone marrow transplantation will be with treatment of specific antibiotics. Granulocytes for interim support may be used if and when the patient appears to have a good chance of endogenous bone marrow recovery. In those instances where the patient's marrow will not recover specific bone marrow transplantation will be used. It does not appear that cryopreserved granulocytes will be available clinically in the immediate future.

DISCUSSION AND CONCLUSIONS

Cryobiology deals with the biochemistry, physiology, anatomy and viability of cells that have undergone cryopreservation. The major effects of cryopreservation are: (1) changes in osmotic pressure; (2) water concentration; and (3) membrane fluidity. Cryopreservation of certain blood cell elements can be aided by the use of cryoprotective agents. These usually easily distribute themselves across the cell membranes and aid in the reduction of the negative effects of the dehydration caused by freezing. At the present time, DMSO is one of the most practical of these agents. A limitation of DMSO for the recipient is that long term use has been associated with some skin and organ changes. The acute effects include its disagreeable odor and possible lysis of red blood cells when not properly washed from the cryopreserved product prior to infusion.

Application of cryobiological techniques has provided red blood cells for a number of years. Platelets are now clinically available and cryopreservation of bone marrow is used at several centers throughout the world. Lymphocytes are easily cryopreserved and although they are not specifically indicated in treatment have utility as reagent cells and possible future clinical applications. Granulocytes do not cryopreserve well under available conditions and no clinical availability of cryopreserved granulocytes is expected in the next five to ten years.

The indications for cryopreserved blood elements other than red cells in the transplantation patient include: (1) cryopreserved platelets for patients with thrombocytopenia and possibly as an aid for host defense mechanisms against certain types of infections; (2) bone marrow transplants for the irradiated or chemotherapeutically treated patient and for long term replacement of granulocyte function in those patients who are granulocytopenic; (3) lymphocytes are useful as reagent cells and possibly for the production of transfer factor; and (4) fresh frozen plasma and cryoprecipitate for protein coagulation problems. The application of cryopreserved blood elements to transplant patients requires evaluation of clinical need so that the proper therapeutic choice is made. Primary concern should be for the immediate correct clinical care of the patient. Other concerns include product availability, viability, cost and potential adverse effects. Understanding and application of evolving cryobiological principles will permit development of methods to provide an expanding array of blood products that may be effectively used to support the transplant patient.

ACKNOWLEDGEMENTS

The invaluable encouragement and assistance of Joyce B. Christopher, Research Specialist, Jim Burkett, Photography Specialist, Emily B. Davidson, Administrative Specialist, all members of the Department of Laboratory Medicine at the Medical University of South Carolina are gratefully acknowledged.

REFERENCES

1. Opelz G, Teresaki PI. Joint Report: International histocompatibility workshop study on renal transplantation. In: Teresaki PI, ed. Histocompatibility testing 1980. UCLA Tissue Typing Laboratory, Los Angeles, Calif., 1980:592–624.
2. Zaroulis CG. Cryopreservation of bone marrow and its clinical application. In: Glassman AB, Umlas J, eds. Cryopreservation of tissue and solid organs for transplantation. AABB 1983:79–90.
3. Wuff JC, Snater TJ, Strob R, et al. Transfusion requirements after HLA identical marrow transplantation in 82 patients with aplastic anemia. Vox Sang 1983;44:366–74.
4. Samson D, Reid C, Chanarin I. Recent advances in haematology. Postgrad Med J 1981;57:139–49.
5. Schiffer CA, Buchholz H, Aisner J, Wolf JH. Frozen autologous platelets in the supportive care of patients with leukemia. Transfusion 1976;16:321–9.
6. Valeri RC. The current state of platelet and granulocyte cryopreservation. Critical Reviews in Clinical Laboratory Sciences 1981;14:21–74.
7. Schiffer C. Platelet cryopreservation. In: Glassman A, Umlas J, eds. Cryopreservation of tissues and solid organs for transplantation. AABB 1983:65–77.
8. Crowe JH, Crowe LM, Mouradian R. Stabilization of biological membranes at low water activities. Cryobiology 1983;20:346–56.
9. Glassman AB, Kawrow AM. Frozen red cells: some cryobiological consideration. American Society of Clinical Pathologists. ASCP Technical Improvement Service 1975;21.
10. Yankee R, Grumet F, Rogentine G. Platelet transfusion therapy-selection of compatible platelet donors for refractory patients by lymphocyte HLA typing. N Engl J Med 1969;281:1208.
11. Lohrmann H, Bull M, Decter J, et al. Platelet transfusion from HLA compatible related donors to alloimmunized patients. Ann Intern Med 1974;80:9.
12. Clift RA, Buckner CD. Supportive measures for patients with aplastic anemia. Clinics in Haematology 1978;7:623–37.
13. Beaujian FR, Leforestier CH, Mannoni P. Clinical and functional studies of platelets frozen in 5% DMSO. Cryo-Letters 1979;1:98–103.
14. Kim BK, Baldine MG. Biochemistry, function and hemostatic effectiveness of frozen human platelets (37904). Proc Soc Exp Biol Med 1974; 145:830–5.
15. Handrin R, Valeri C. Improved viability of previously frozen platelets. Blood 1972;40:509–13.
16. Melaragno A, Abdu W, Katchis R, Vecchione J, Valeri C. Cryopreservation of platelets isolated with the IBM 2997 blood cell separator: a rapid and simplified approach. Vox Sang 1982;43:321–6.
17. Rowe A, Lenny L. Platelets. In: Karow A, Pegg D, eds. Organ preservation for transplantation. New York and Basel: Marcel Dekker, Inc. 1981:335–54.
18. Liu PI, Ogawa M, Crook L, Ochia R, Upshur JK. Proliferative function of cadaveric bone marrow cells. Am J of Hematol 1978;5:145–50.
19. Iscove JS, Senn S, Till JE, McCulloch EA. Colony formation by normal and leukemic human marrow cells in culture: effect of conditioned medium from human leukocytes. Blood 1971;37:1–5.

20. Ogawa M, Parmley RT, Bank HL, Spicer SS. Human marrow erytropoiesis in culture. I. Characterization of methylcellulose colony assay. Blood 1976;48:407–17.
21. Liu PI, Poon Kc, Liu SS, Crook L. Cryopreservation of human cadaveric bone cells. Cryobiology 1980;17:419–23.
22. Liu PI, Poon KC, Hong CC, Crook L, Liu SS, Mitsuoki E. In vitro and in vivo assessment of the viability of cryopreserved postmortem murine bone marrow cells. Ann Clin Lab Sci 1980;10:165–8.
23. McClave P, Ramsay N, Kersey J. Bone marrow transplantation at the university of Minnesota. Minn Med 1982;65:351–4.
24. Herzig GP. Autologous bone marrow transplantation in cancer therapy. Prog in Hematol 1981;12:1–23.
25. Dicke KA, Vellekoop L, Spitzer G, Zander AR, Schell F, Verma DS. Autologous bone marrow transplantation in neoplasia. In: Gale RP, Fox CF, eds. Biology of Bone Marrow Transplantation 1980:159–65.
26. American Red Cross. Advances in immunology: blood cell antigens and bone marrow transplantation. XV Annual Scientific Symposium, May 1983, Washington, D.C.
27. Conrad ME. An introduction to bone marrow transplantation: leukemia and aplastic disease — new solutions for old problems. Ala J of Med Sci 1981;18:231–2.
28. Glassman AB, Bennet CE. Cryopreservation of human lymphocytes: a brief review and evaluation of an automated liquid nitrogen freezer. Transfusion 1979;19:178–81.
29. Golub SH. Cryopreservation of human lymphocytes. In: Bloom BR, David JR, eds. In vitro methods in cell-mediated and tumor immunity. New York: Academic Press 1976:731–5.
30. Glassman AB, Christopher JC. Effect of cryopreservation on lymphocyte markers as evaluated by monoclonal antibodies. Transfusion 1983;23:426.
31. Appelbaum FR, Oldham RK. Cryopreservation of human lymphocyte function. In: Proceedings of The Haemonectics Research Institute. Advanced Component Seminar. Massachusetts: Haemonetics Research Institute, 1978.
32. Vogler WR. Organ preservation for transplantation. In: Karow AM, Pegg DE, eds. Granulocytes and lymphocytes. New York and Basel: Marcel Dekker, Inc. 1981:323–33.

DISCUSSION

Moderators: G. Opelz, D.W. van Bekkum

W.G. Ho (UCLA, Los Angeles):

Dr. Glassman, with regard to the utility of the cryopreserved platelets, I think the technique that you have described is a feasible one. With regard to the clinical application, I wonder what the use of cryopreserved platelets actually will be. The reason for this is that I can think of two situations where platelets will be needed at a very frequent rate, that is in support of patients undergoing bone-marrow transplantation, and in support of patients undergoing intensive chemotherapy for diseases which are mainly acute leukemias. With regard to the bone-marrow transplantation, there really would be no need for cryopreserved platelets, for as long as an HLA identical sibling is available fresh HLA matched platelets can be used.

In the support of patients with leukemia, I think there is a limited need for cryopreserved platelets in that respect. One, because the actual period during which the patients will need such platelets is limited to the time that those patients are in aplastic phase of their treatment. Generally, this is about three weeks. One can actually support the patient with regular non-cryopreserved platelets, until they start to make their own platelets.

In the event patients are alloimmunized and do not get a good result from regular platelets, then from family members who are at least compatible. HLA matched platelets are generally available. Those platelets apparently seem to be just as useful as fully matched autologous platelets. Therefore, the actual need for cryopreserved platelets is something about which I am in doubt.

A.B. Glassman (Charleston, U.S.A.):

Thank you, Dr. Ho. I agree with all of your comments. It is one of the reasons why I put a question mark as to whether there will be need for the application of cryopreserved platelets. Indeed, I think that it is an expensive way and those platelets do not function very well. One would need a long period of time to collect sufficient autologous platelets to freeze them so that you could treat every other day, or every two days, for a period of time when a patient is suffering from the effects of acute chemo or radiation therapy.

So I agree entirely. The methods for cryopreservation of platelets extend back into the early 1970's. From a historical standpoint, if a good method is around and if there had been a need, I think that more of our Blood Banks would be supplying cryopreserved platelets. So, from a historical standpoint, your point is borne out as well.

B. Löwenberg (Rotterdam, The Netherlands):

Dr. Glassman, you showed that there was a decreased increment following transfusion of cryopreserved platelets, and also a loss of function. Could you indicate what the ultimate recovery is, if you take into account these two phenomena?

A.B. Glassman:

That is a complex question. If one examines the decreased increment, that is about 60% for liquid platelets versus 40% plus or minus in the cryopreserved platelets, and one looks at the decreased length of time that the bleeding time is corrected, I would say that the effectiveness is down to 25 or 30% of what the effectiveness of a liquid preserved platelet would be. That would be an estimate.

P.C. Das (Groningen, The Netherlands):

Professor Gips, I refer to the recent consensus meeting on liver transplantation held at the National Institute of Health, in America, where the Groningen Group has presented a constructive document. With regard to such measured transplant operations, what is the summary of this consensus? Secondly, what is your view or advice on this subject?

C.H. Gips (Groningen, The Netherlands):

The summary of the consensus meeting was that liver transplantation is a treatment modality, that should not be regarded anymore as some kind of experimental medicine. There should be a limited number of centres only, because of the complexity of this type of medicine and, although it is not to be regarded as experimental any longer, there is still much to be learned. There are at present four centres in the United States and Europe. These have been limited by the lack of resources, but will eventually increase in number.

However, the main issue is that liver transplantation should be regarded as a treatment modality, and that it should be funded.

F. Mercuriali (Milan, Italy):

Dr. Hendriks, you said that DRw6 positive transplants are prednisone resistant and that the outcome of the graft can be improved by treating the patients with ATG. My question is: Has this been given prophylactically, or just for treating rejection episodes? In the case of prophylactic therapy, could you indicate the length of the therapy and the dosage?

G.F.J. Hendriks (Leiden, The Netherlands):

Acute rejections were treated in two different ways. In one group of patients the oral dose of prednison was raised to 200 mg/day and tapered in 3- or 5-day periods to 100, 75, 50, 40, 30 and 25 mg. Intravenous steroid pulses were not used. In the other group acute rejections were treated with a three-weeks course of rabbit antithymocyte-globulin (RATG). The initial dose was 4 mg/kg and additional doses were between 2 and 7 mg/kg depending on the peripheral T_3-cell level that we tried to keep between 50 and 150/mm^3. The prednisone dose was not raised in these patients except for the addition of 50 mg prednisolone to the first and 25 mg to each following RATG infusion to avoid acute side effects. If the patients experienced a second rejection episode or if the first rejection responded insufficiently to treatment, the alternative treatment was given.

R.A.F. Krom (Groningen, The Netherlands):

Dr. Hendriks, the DRw6 item is fascinating. You referred to your data from the kidneys transplanted. However, I wonder, whether those data are available from other organs like livers or bone marrow, corneas, hearts, or is it specific to the kidneys themselves? Can you give any correlation with respect to other organ grafting so far? It could be done easily in large centres where liver transplants are performed. One needs a large group of recipients, because the frequency of DRw6 is about 25%. So, in a group of 100 transplants, one will have approximately 25 donors which are DRw6 positive.

G.F.J. Hendriks:

No data were published so far, concerning "the DRw6 phenomenon" in recipients of liver and heart transplants. By performing HLA-A, -B and especially HLA-DR typings of those recipients and their organ donors, large centres would be able to analyse their data with respect to MHC-restricted immune responsiveness and non-responsiveness. In centres where corneal transplants are performed only recipients of vascularised corneas should be analysed.

R.A.F. Krom:

Unfortunately, in liver transplantation there are many other factors where donor-recipient combinations fail. You have heard from Dr. Gips that even selection is important. I can imagine that looking at the results with a high yield of successful transplants, there must be some data in heart transplantation about DRw6.

G. Opelz (Heidelberg, FRG):

You would need quite a number of patients to perform a good analysis. Dr. Ford told us about a very interesting and novel immunological phenomenon that does not require T cells, does not require B cells, does not require immunoglobulin. As an immunologist, one begins to wonder whether there is any immunology involved at all. Dr. Ford, is there any effect of immunosuppressive drugs on this type of phenomenon? What if you treat the animals with cyclophosphamide?

W.L. Ford (Manchester, U.K.):

One observation that brings the rejection of allogeneic lymphocytes into the realm of immunology is that rodents made tolerant as neonates by the injection of allogeneic bone marrow not only fail to reject skin grafts but also fail to reject lymphocytes from the specific donor type. This experiment has been done in Bainbridge's laboratory* and also in Barbara Heslop's laboratory**. This mechanism of allogeneic lymphocyte rejection begins within 30 minutes of cell transfer so a very rapid distinction between "self" and "non-self" is implied. If lymphocytes are not involved it becomes urgently necessary to identify the cell type that is responsible. The main candidates are macrophages, dendritic cells and NK cells. Allogeneic lymphocyte rejection is resistant to high doses of whole-body irradiation*** although the rejection is transiently impaired two weeks after the irradiation. Blockade of the mononuclear phagocytic system does not seem to inhibit rejection. Barbara Heslop and her colleagues have recently found that cyclosporin A and hydrocortisone have no effect on this mechanism and cyclophosphamide impairs it only slightly.

D.W. van Bekkum (Rijswijk, The Netherlands):

Dr. Hendriks, you mentioned that the number of tumors that developed in kidney transplant patients is larger when you have more AB0 mismatches. Is it possible to distinguish immuno-genetically between the donor-recipient relationship itself? Could it be that patients with two or three mismatches receive higher dosages of immunosuppressive agents? Have you distinguished these two factors?

G.F.J. Hendriks:

This paper was published in Cancer****. The correlation between the number of HLA-A, -B mismatches, the dosis of corticosteroids, and tumor incidence was not analysed. However, a significantly higher incidence of tumors was observed in recipients of necrokidneys compared with related kidneys. This might indicate a correlation between the three parameters mentioned above. Another interesting observation was the significant over-representation of recipients with chronic interstitial nephritis.

* Bainbridge DR. Eliminations of allogeneic lymphocytes by mice. Immunol Rev 1983;73:5–34.
** Heslop BF, McNeilage J. Natural cytotoxicity: Early killing of allogeneic lymphocytes in rats. Immunol Rev 1983;73:35–52.
*** Rolstad B, Ford WL. The rapid elimination of allogeneic lymphocytes: Relationship to establish mechanisms of immunity and to lymphocyte traffic. Immunol Rev 1983;73:87–114.
**** Birkeland SA. Malignant tumors in renal transplant patients; the scandia transplant material. Cancer 1983;51:1571–5.

G. Opelz:

We are conducting a prospective, multicentre, world-wide study in which we follow currently over 80,000 patients. We are looking at the type and dose of immunosuppression, the genetic background, and tumor development. It will be a couple of years before we have the answers.

D.W. van Bekkum:

Dr. Hendriks, what happens if you treat the patients with cyclosporin A instead of immunosuppressives and prednisolon?

G.F.J. Hendriks:

The data of 250 renal transplant patients treated with CyA could be analysed. These patients were transplanted in centres collaborating in Eurotransplant. The group of recipients at risk after one year is small, and the data are preliminary. In this group however, the same beneficial effect of HLA-A, -B and DR matching was observed, compared with other studies performed in the period before CyA was used. This beneficial effect is absent during the first six months after transplantation, but emerges at twelve months postoperatively. Whether or not a conversion to conservative treatment is involved, remains to be analysed.

G. Opelz:

I can support this. We have now data on nearly 1,000 cyclosporin A treated patients and there is an effect of HLA matching: cyclosporin does not overcome the effect of matching.

II. SUPPORTIVE HEMOTHERAPY

IMMUNE MODULATION ASPECTS OF BLOOD TRANSFUSION IN TRANSPLANTATION PRACTICE*

G.G. Persijn

GENERAL PREFACE

There are many ways to alter the immune response of a recipient to an organ graft. Sofar, the most successful approaches in renal transplantation are matching of donors and recipients for the HLA-A, -B and -DR antigens, the use of immunosuppressive drugs and pretransplant blood transfusions. The latter factor has received considerable attention since Opelz and Terasaki in 1973 (1) reported that kidney graft recipients who never had received blood transfusions prior to transplantation had a very poor kidney graft survival. Since then, many different protocols have been designed for experimental and clinical studies to investigate the role of pretransplant blood transfusions in renal transplantation.

The majority of the reports demonstrate a significant benefit of pretransplant blood transfusions on renal allograft survival. However, there are some significant discrepancies among the published results. Explanations of the (precise) mechanism whereby blood transfusions modulate the immune response towards a kidney graft are mainly speculative.

Thus, although much work has been performed in an attempt to unravel the precise role of blood transfusions in renal transplantation, much remains unclear.

A critical review of the available data in the world literature as well as our own experience in The Netherlands about how and why blood transfusions act in modulating the immune response is presented.

INTRODUCTION

In the early days of regular hemodialysis renal patients were liberally transfused. Since the end of the sixties this policy has changed which is shown by a decrease in the median number of blood transfusions administered to the dialysis patients awaiting kidney transplantation (2). This change resulted from the realization that dialysis patients could be well maintained without regular blood transfusions by using the more sophisticated smaller artificial kidneys and without pretransplant bilateral nefrectomy. Furthermore, the restricted blood transfusion policy would reduce the risk of

* This work was in part supported by the Dutch Foundation for Medical Research (FUNGO) which is subsidized by the Dutch Organization for the Advancement of Pure Research (ZWO), the J.A. Cohen Institute for Radiopathology and Radiation Protection (IRS) and the Kuratorium für Heimdialyse, Neu-Isenburg, Germany.

hepatitis and the induction of anti-HLA antibody production. Increased immunization of the potential transplant recipient was associated with lower kidney graft survival (3). Besides these aspects, sensitized kidney patients have a longer waiting time for a cadaver kidney transplant and, in some cases, may not be able to receive a transplant at all due to cytotoxic antibodies.

Consequently, many dialysis doctors avoided to transfuse potential kidney transplant candidates. This policy led to discomfort in some patients who had to live with very low hematocrit levels which did handicap them in many ways. Especially the bilaterally nefrectomized patients. In this way a group of never transfused patients awaiting a cadaveric renal transplant was "created". Paradoxically, to what had been expected kidney graft survival in this particular group of patients was not improved by avoiding blood transfusions and thus immunization. On the contrary, kidney graft survival times were worse if compared to graft survival in the transfused group of recipients. Opelz et al. in 1973 were the first investigators who drew attention to this particular fact (1).

From a historical point of view it is interesting that others already had suggested that blood transfusions did not detrimentally influence kidney graft survival (4,5). Since that initial report many centres were able to demonstrate retrospectively a beneficial influence of pretransplant blood transfusions on kidney allograft survival in man. Prospective studies in monkeys (6) and dogs (7) had provided unequivocal evidence that pretransplant third party blood transfusions improve the fate of kidney allografts from unrelated donors.

ACCEPTANCE OF THE BLOOD TRANSFUSION EFFECT

Since in 1973 Opelz et al. (1) originally reported on the beneficial effect of pretransplant blood transfusion on cadaveric kidney allograft survival, numerous additional reports have been published. The majority of them agree that blood transfusions do have a beneficial effect on cadaveric renal allograft survival. The Oxford group initially did not see a beneficial influence of pretransplant blood transfusion on kidney allograft survival (8). However, later studies could demonstrate a beneficial effect. It has to be stressed that the graft survival in their non-transfused patients is rather high as compared to other centres (9).

Experimental studies in animal models, like the Rhesus monkey, clearly have demonstrated a positive influence of pretransplant blood transfusion on kidney allograft survival (6,10).

The overall conclusion is that pretransplant transfusions have a beneficial effect on cadaveric kidney graft survival. However, no general agreement has been reached on the influence of different variables such as the exact number of transfusions; the composition of the transfusate and the risk of sensitization; the time interval between transfusion and transplantation; the use of HLA-matched blood transfusions; the use of blood transfusions in recipients of a related transplant; the effect of transfusions on subsequent transplants and finally, the influence of blood transfusions given to the kidney donor. In addition the mechanisms, underlying the beneficial effect of blood transfusion on kidney graft survival, remain unknown and speculative.

The state of affairs of some of the above mentioned parameters will be described.

NUMBER OF TRANSFUSIONS

Survey of the literature

There is no unanimity concerning a beneficial dose-related transfusion effect. Sometimes, studies from the same centre disagreed with their own previous reports (11–13). Some reports showed that even a single blood transfusion was as effective as many transfusions (14–16). Other investigators observed that the best graft survival was obtained with 2 or 3 units of blood (9,17–19) while others demonstrated the maximum effect on graft survival with up to 5 units of blood (20–22). Also the results, obtained during the 8th International Histocompatibility Workshop, did not give a definite answer on this point (23). In this international multicentre study there seemed to be a dose-effect of transfusions. Indeed, all the different subgroups of patients according to the number of transfusions had a significantly better graft survival as compared to the graft survival in non-transfused recipients. However, graft survival in the various transfused groups was not statistically different from each other. This observation was confirmed in a prospective study too (24,25). Nevertheless, the best survival was achieved in the group of recipients who had received more than 20 blood transfusions.

PROSPECTIVE STUDY

In the Netherlands it was decided that never-transfused and/or nulliparous kidney patients awaiting a cadaveric kidney transplant should prospectively be transfused with one unit of washed ABO-identical blood. Another group of never-transfused and/or nulliparous patients was given 1 or 3 units of cotton-wool filtered blood. Blood was not longer stored than 3 days and considered to be fresh. It was found unethical to continue transplanting non-transfused kidney patients. Consequently, a prospective non-transfused control group was not available for this study.

The aims of this protocol were to investigate the influence of different variables such as the number of transfusions, the compostion of the transfusate, the time interval between transfusion and transplantation and the HLA-type of the blood transfusion and kidney donor. The choice to use washed erythrocytes was based on the results in the retrospective study. Besides this, the risk of immunization against HLA-antigens was low, especially when 1 unit was given (26). By washing the blood and removing the buffy-coat about 40-60% of the leukocytes are removed.

RESULTS OF THE PROSPECTIVE STUDY

Table I shows the relevant data of the recipients in this prospective study. All patients, who were transfused according to this protocol but who later required additional transfusions prior to transplantation for medical reasons were excluded from this study. Most of the serum samples tested after the transfusion of these patients showed no detectable lymphocytotoxic antibody activity. In 2 cases very weak activity amounting to approximately 5% kill above background developed. This activity had disappeared in subsequent serum samples. All patients received 16 blood transfusions, mostly leukocyte-free blood (cotton-wool filtration method) during transplantation (27).

Table I. Profile of the prospective study (1977–1980).

Number of transfusions	Composition of transfusate	Number of patients		Age in years	Hemodialysis period in months	Average HLA-mismatch kidney donor-recipient (HLA-A and -B)
		male	female			
1	leukocyte poor	31	9	16-56 (36)*	3-68 (19)**	1.6
1	leukocyte free	6	-	31-56 (36.5)*	3-21 (10)**	1.7
3	leukocyte free	3	3	16-50 (37.5)*		

* The mean age.
** The mean hemodialysis period.

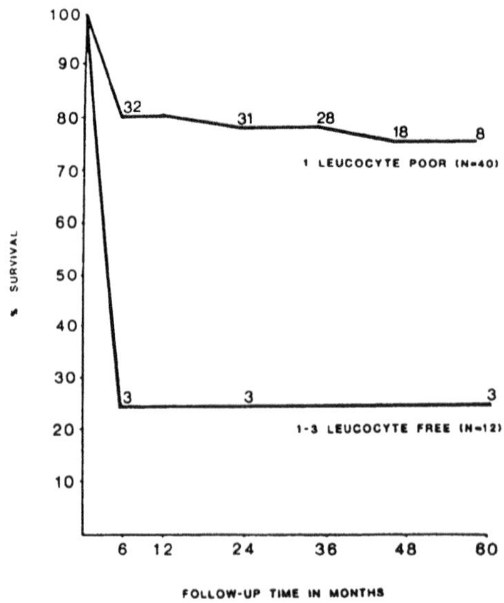

Figure 1. The 5-year kidney graft survival results in the prospective blood transfusion study in previously non-transfused recipients. The upper line represents kidney graft survival of a group of 40 patients who have been prospectively transfused with 1 transfusion of leukocyte-poor blood. The lower curve shows the kidney graft survival in 12 patients who have been prospectively been transfused with 1–3 transfusions of leukocyte-free blood. The difference in graft survival between the two groups is significant p=0.01).

Figure 1 shows that kidney graft survival in these 40 patients is 78% after 5 years which is significantly better than 28% graft survival in our retrospective non-transfused group (N=74, $p < 0.001$; this curve not shown). The results of this prospective blood transfusion study – although not randomized in the real sense, but close to it – confirms the beneficial effect of 1 pretransplant blood transfusion observed in our retrospective study (28).

Other authors have shown in single-centre studies also an improvement in kidney graft survival in patients who had received one or very few blood transfusions before transplantation (8,14,29,30).

THE COMPOSITION OF THE TRANSFUSATE

Survey of the literature

Considerable disagreement exists concerning the composition of the transfusate. Most clinicians attempt to avoid possible sensitization by blood transfusions because of the poorer graft survival obtained in recipients with lymphocytotoxic antibodies. Russell (31) recommended a minimum number of blood transfusions from which the leukocytes have been either removed or killed by freezing. However, the literature shows no general agreement on the effect of frozen blood on kidney allograft survival. Opelz et al. (32) and Säfwenberg et al. (33) have reported that frozen blood is ineffective in improving cadaveric kidney graft survival. Contrarily, other investigators could demonstrate that frozen blood was as effective as other blood products such as whole blood, packed cells of leukocyte-poor blood (29, 34–37). This beneficial effect of frozen blood should be dependent on the method used for freezing, as mentioned by Fuller et al. (38). The deglycerolization method by agglomeration should be preferred to the deglycerolization method by centrifugal washing.

Still, the beneficial transfusion effect on kidney allograft survival was mostly noticed when the patients had received whole blood or leukocyte-poor blood transfusions (1,9,14,17,19,30,39,40).

To avoid the detrimental effect of sensitizing the potential kidney transplant recipient and to save the beneficial influence of pretransplant blood transfusion, several prospective blood transfusion protocols have been designed. Some approaches are worth mentioning here, namely the protocol introduced by Nubé et al. (41). They proposed to transfuse potential kidney graft recipients with 2 or 3 units of HLA-A and -B compatible leukocyte poor blood transfusions. Thus, the potential transplant candidates received blood transfusions without HLA-A and -B mismatches. Graft survival in this "pretreated" group of patients was 86% at 2 years, thus not significantly different from graft survival in the group of patients prospectively transfused with single random blood transfusion.

Albert et al. (42) had a similar approach, although here, the recipients were transfused with HLA-A and -B matched leukocyte-poor blood. In this study it was impossible to transfuse all patients with HLA-A and -B compatible blood. Thus, there remained differences for the HLA-A and -B antigens between blood transfusion donor and kidney recipient. In this study, no beneficial effect could be demonstrated. Furthermore, quite a few patients developed anti-HLA antibodies.

Very recently the Leuven group published a Letter in the New England Journal of Medicine that they were unable to demonstrate a beneficial effect of HLA-A and -B compatible blood transfusions on renal allograft survival. However, this statement was based on only 4 patients of which 2 lost their grafts. Another 26 patients, who had received previously random blood transfusion and later HLA-A and -B compatible blood transfusions, had all functioning grafts at 1 year (43).

Also recently, Borleffs et al. (44) have observed a beneficial effect of pure platelet transfusion on kidney graft survival in the Rhesus monkey. This elegant approach might be of clinical advantage because pure platelet transfusions do not induce leukocyte antibody formation. However, a very preliminar report on clinical results did not clearly support the findings in the Rhesus monkeys (A. Ting, personal communication).

RESULTS OF THE PROSPECTIVE STUDY

The blood transfusion protocol introduced in The Netherlands in 1977 included also a group of non-transfused patients who were transfused with 1 to 3 units of cotton-wool filtered blood. With this technique the fresh blood is almost totally depleted from leukocytes and is called leukocyte-free blood (27). Most of the dialysis specialists, who discussed the transfusion protocol with their patients, favoured the donation of only one transfusion. Table I gives the relevant information of this group. All patients received transfusions of leukocyte-free blood varying from 1 to 4 units, during the operation.

Figure 1 shows that kidney graft survival in this group of recipients is 33% after 5 years. This is significantly different from the survival in the group prospectively given 1 unit of leukocyte-poor blood ($p=0.01$). The survival in the group pretreated prospectively with 1 or 3 units of leukocyte-free blood does not differ significantly from the 28% graft survival at 5 years in our retrospective nontransfused group (this curve not shown).

A few remarks should be made. Firstly, none of the patients in this prospective study needed a blood transfusion. The blood transfusion was given really prospectively. Secondly, during this protocol it turned out already quickly, that patients transfused with 1 or 3 leukocyte-free blood transfusions rejected their kidney very rapidly. This observation prompted the nephrologists to switch to the "leukocyte-poor" protocol. This explains why only 12 patients are in the leukocyte-free group. Thirdly, the 3 patients with a functioning graft are all from the same transplant centre. Interestingly, investigation learned that the blood used for preparation of leukocyte-free blood in this centre was already one week old which is against the prescription. It is suspected that leukocyte fragments are not removed from one week old blood by cotton-wool filtration. This might explain the "transfusion effect" in these 3 patients.

TIMING OF THE TRANSFUSION

Survey of the literature

The role of the duration of the interval between blood transfusion and transplantation is still uncertain. Buy-Quang et al. (14) have reported that a better graft survival was achieved when transfusions had occurred within 6 months before grafting. More recently, Hourmant et al. (17) from the same group have stated that the transfusion effect was strongest if the last unit was given within 3 months of transplantation. Also, Werner-Favre et al. (45) and Fauchet et al. (146) have found the same correlation. However, the latter showed also that all 8 patients who had received the last transfusion more than 12 months before transplantation had a functioning graft at 1 year.

Yet, many other clinical data including those of the International Workshop study did not support these findings (16,19,23,28,47).

One of the main problems in cadaveric renal transplantation is that one never knows when the patient will be transplanted. This consideration has led to prospective protocols in which the patient will receive peri- or peroperative blood transfusion. Thus, blood transfusion given within 6 hours before (peri) or during (per) transplantation.

The NIH-Registry Report (48), Stiller et al. (49), Hunsicker et al. (35) and Williams et al. (9) demonstrated that transfusions given to non-transfused recipients at the time of transplantation have a beneficial effect on kidney graft survival. Again, others, including ourselves, have not been able to confirm this (13,46,50–52).

Recently, Fassbinder et al. (53) showed that 2 units of buffy-coat rich erythrocytes, one given 4 hours and the other given 1 hour before transplantation, gave a 74% kidney graft survival at 2 years in a group of never-transfused patients. A similar transfusion protocol in previously transfused patients resulted in a 72% graft survival at 2 years. Therefore, they concluded that blood transfusions with sufficient leukocytes given peri-operatively have a beneficial effect on kidney graft survival too.

The different protocols used in the different centres make it very difficult to draw firm conclusions on the effect of peri- or peroperative blood transfusion (54).

RESULTS OF THE PROSPECTIVE STUDY

The time between transfusion and transplantation in the Dutch group of 40 patients who received prospectively 1 unit of leukocyte-poor blood varied from 21 days to 1108 days (mean: 251 days). A clearcut correlation between the time of transfusion and kidney graft outcome was not observed (table II). On the other hand, 6 out of 8 transplants into patients receiving leukocyte-free blood within 200 days before transplantation failed within 3 months.

Table II. Time interval between blood transfusion and kidney transplantation in the different prospectively transfused groups.

Time interval (days)	Function/total at 1 year	
	Leukocyte-poor	Leukocyte-free
0–100	10/12	1/5
101–200	8/11	1/6
201–300	4/4	-
301–400	5/6	1/1
401–500	2/3	-
501	3/4	-

OTHER FACTORS

Besides the already described parameters which seem to play an important role in the effect or pretransplant blood transfusions on kidney allograft survival many other factors seems to be relevant too. Reviewing the literature provides an enormous amount of such, sometimes conflicting, factors.

Joysey et al. (55) found that the beneficial effect of transfusions was restricted to patients of blood group O. This finding has been confirmed by Bore et al. (56). However, other did not find such an association with blood group O (39,57).

Festenstein et al. (58) showed that a beneficial effect of pretransplant blood transfusion was only apparent in patients with well HLA-A and -B matched kidneys. No difference was found in graft survival in recipients who received a poorly HLA-A and -B matched kidney whether they were transfused or not. Also Spees et al. (37) found that the better the HLA-A and -B match between donor and transfused recipient, the better the transplant survival.

Uldall et al. (47) reported that the best kidney graft survival was obtained in transfused patients who received an HLA-B locus identical kidney. Williams et al. (9) did not find any interaction between the transfusion effect and the degree of donor-recipient matching for the HLA-A and -B antigens. However, when HLA-DR matching was taken into account, he stated that a safe procedure to overcome the risk of transfusion is to ensure that the non-transfused recipient receives a well HLA-DR matched kidney.

The International Workshop Study showed a consistent correlation of HLA-A and -B matching and graft survival in non-transfused patients (23). The correlation was weaker in patients who had received only a few blood transfusions, where as there was no correlation in patients with more than 10 transfusions. The effect of matching is larger outweighed by multiple blood transfusions.

Fehrman et al. (59) noticed only a transfusion effect in male recipients, while no such an effect was seen in female recipients. Solheim (52) found also a more pronounced effect of transfusions in males than in females. Williams et al. (9) could not demonstrate such a correlation.

Guttmann et al. (60) showed a highly significant correlation between the length of dialysis and the number of transfusions. Fehrman et al. (40) revealed that graft survival was positively correlated with pretransplant dialysis, more strongly than with transfusions. However, Buy-Quang et al. (14) stated that duration of dialysis was less important than blood transfusions and pregnancies, which was also observed by Solheim (52).

Alexandre et al. (22) reported that very superior graft survival was obtained in transfused recipients who were treated with ALS or ATG. This observation was confirmed by Spees et al. (37).

The transfusion effect was most optimal in patients who did not develop lymphocytotoxic antibodies, as found by Sirchia et al. (30). Also, others have reported the same findings (1), while Werner-Favre et al. (45) could not show any influence of antilymphocytotoxic or anti-B cell antibodies on kidney graft survival.

Significantly better graft survival was observed by Andrus et al. (61) in multitransfused recipients who remained free of cytomegaly-infection.

No effect of autologous blood transfusions on kidney allograft survival was seen by Säfwenberg et al. (33).

A reduced transfusion effect was noticed in black recipients of a cadaveric kidney graft, by Spees et al. (37).

Finally, the role of previous pregnancies on kidney allograft survival. Fauchet et al. (45) have suggested an additive effect of transfusions and previous pregnancies. Also, other investigators have stated that a pregnancy had much the same effect on kidney graft survival as blood transfusions (14,17,62).

Analysis of the Dutch data showed that 15 never-transfused female recipients who had been previously pregnant had a 50% graft survival at 1 year. This is a 20% improvement as compared to graft survival in patients who never had received blood transfusions nor had been pregnant.

Solheim (52) demonstrated that identical graft survival was obtained in non-transfused women with previous pregnancies as non-transfused women without pregnancies. Also, Opelz et al. (63) found no evidence that pregnancies improved the outcome of cadaveric grafts substantially.

MECHANISMS

The mechanism by which blood transfusions improve renal allograft survival is still unknown and remains speculative. Several hypotheses have been proposed such as a selection hypothesis and a protection hypothesis.

According to the selection hypothesis, patients who respond with high levels of cytotoxic antibodies, the socalled "high responders" are selected out by the cross-match. They will be never transplanted unless a fully-matched, i.e., HLA-A, -B and -C identical donor-kidney becomes available. Patients who do not produce antibodies after many blood transfusions are the so-called "non" or "low responders" (32). Probably, they can be transplanted with any donor kidney. Against this hypothesis is that 1 single blood transfusion gives already an improvement of graft survival (28). After administration of 1 single blood transfusion, no good division can be made into low and high responders (26). Besides this, graft survival is enhanced by blood transfusions in patients with all levels of cytotoxic antibodies (21). Furthermore, the selection hypothesis does not explain the reported beneficial effect of per-operative blood transfusions either (9,35,49).

Another approach has been developed to distinguish (hemo)dialysis patients as responders or non-responders, i.e., the use of the quantitative dinitrochlorobenzene (DNCB) skin test (36). Studies, in which blood transfusions given to such patients, interact with the DNCB-reactivity are under way.

The second possibility is the protection hypothesis, which is based on the idea that antigens present in the donor blood induce enhancing antibody formation. Ferrara et al. (64) have shown that repeated stimulation with small doses of HLA-antigen induces a state of unresponsiveness in man. This phenomenon has been reported by other investigators in experimental animal models after multiple blood transfusions (65). The nature of these enhancing antibodies is still unknown. MLC-blocking antibodies, cold B-cell antibodies, anti Ia-like or anti HLA-DR antibodies and anti-idiotypic antibodies have been suggested as enhancing antibodies (16,45,66–68).

Recently, anti-idiotypic antibodies could be shown only in the serum of patients who had received pretransplant blood transfusion and in female patients during pregnancy (69). In transfused patients these anti-idiotypic antibodies were demonstrable only in patients with functioning kidney grafts and not in patients who had rejected the graft (70).

Another explanation for this protection mechanism might be the induction of suppressor cells after blood transfusions (71). Increased suppressor cell function has been reported 3 weeks after the administration of 2 units of packed red cells in chronic hemodialysis patients (72). Also, marked suppression of cellular immunity in never-transfused hemodialysis patients have been observed after transfusion of washed erythrocytes (73). This phenomenon was not observed when autologous blood was given.

Evidence has been demonstrated, in an experimental dog model, that blood transfusions led to a macrophage blockade which leads to improved renal allograft survival as suggested by Keown and Descamps (74).

Finally, Goulmy et al. (75) have demonstrated that donor cell specific mediated lymphlysis (CML) did not occur in 70% of the recipients with a good functioning cadaveric kidney graft. All patients who had rejected their graft were CML-reactive. In only 1 case out of 7 CML-non responders studied, suppressor cells were shown to be present. All patients in this study had received 1 or more blood transfusions. A possible explanation for this specific CML-non reactivity could be that the specific anti-donor cytotoxic clones of the effector cells are eliminated by anti-idiotypic antibodies or by absorption in the graft.

In conclusion, most of the work done in animals as well as in humans suggests that unspecific suppressor cells are responsible for the graft prolongation effect of pretransplant blood transfusion. However, the possibility remains that there might be different phases and steps caused by blood transfusions which results in the acceptance of a donor organ.

Maybe, that the use of monoclonal antibodies, such as the OKT-sera, in monitoring renal patients after the administration of blood transfusions will give a definite answer in the near future.

CONCLUSIONS

Pretransplant blood transfusions have a beneficial effect on cadaveric kidney graft survival. Some evidence exists for a similar "transfusion effect" on living related transplants, especially in the group of patients who receive a haplo-identical related kidney.

The optimal number of blood transfusions to obtain an effect is still under discussion although some centres, including our own, have observed this effect already after only 1 or a few blood transfusions. A reduced number of transfusions, especially of whole blood, has been recommended. In our opinion the best policy would be to give 1 single transfusion of leukocyte poor blood to the recipient.

The composition of the transfusion appears to be important. Viable leukocytes into the transfusate seem to be a pre-requisite to induce a "transfusion effect". Very recently, pure platelets seem to be very effective in prolonging kidney graft survival in the Rhesus monkey (44). What the clinical relevance will be has to be investigated in well designed protocols.

Some data indicate that it would be ideal to transfuse HLA-A and -B matched leukocyte poor blood to the kidney patient.

The optimal time-interval might be within 200 days before transplantation. Peri- or peroperative transfusions might also be beneficial, but this is still controversial. Anyhow, no detrimental effects of peri- or peroperative transfusions on kidney graft outcome have been reported sofar.

Finally, the mechanism underlying the blood transfusion effect in renal transplantation is still unclear. Although much of the work done in humans suggests that non-specific suppressor cells are responsible for this effect, other possibilities like the production of enhancing antibodies, antigen-antibody complexes or anti-idiotypic antibodies or the induction of specific anti-donor cytotoxic clones cannot be excluded.

REFERENCES

1. Opelz G, Mickey MR, Terasaki PI. Blood transfusions and unresponsiveness to HL-A. Transplantation 1973;16:649–54.
2. Hooff JP van, Kalff MW, Poelgeest AE van, Persijn GG, Rood JJ van. Blood transfusions and kidney transplantation. Transplantation 1976;22: 306–7.
3. Hooff JP van, Schippers HMA, Steen GJ van der, Rood JJ van. Efficacy of HL-A matching in Eurotransplant. Lancet 1972;ii:1385–8.
4. Michielsen, P. Hémodialyse et transplantation rénale. EDTA Proc 1979;3: 162–4.
5. Dossetor JB, MacKinnon KJ, Gault MH, Maclean LD. Cadaver kidney transplants. Transplantation 1967;5:844–53.
6. Es AA van, Marquet RL, Rood JJ van, Kalff MW, Balner H. Blood transfusions induce prolonged kidney allograft survival in Rhesus monkeys. Lancet 1977;i:506–9.
7. Obertop H, Bijnen AB, Niessen G.J.C.M., Joling P. The influence of number and timing of pretransplant blood transfusion on the beneficial effect of renal allograft survival in immunosuppressed dogs. Eur Surg Res 1981;13:21–4.
8. Morris PJ, Oliver D, Bishop M, et al. Results from a new renal transplantation unit. Lancet 1978;ii:1353–6.
9. Williams GM, Ting A, Cullen PR, Morris PH. Transfusions: Their influence on human renal graft survival. Transplant Proc 1979;11:175–8.
10. Borleffs JCC, Marquet RL, Balner H. Pretransplant blood transfusions have an additive positive effect on kidney graft prognosis in D/DR-matched Rhesus monkeys. Transplantation 1981;32:48–50.
11. Opelz G, Terasaki PI. Enhancement of kidney graft survival by blood transfusions. Transplant Proc 1977;9:121–2.
12. Opelz G, Terasaki PI, Graver B, et al. Correlation between number of pretransplant blood transfusions and kidney graft survival. Transplant Proc 1979;9:145–7.
13. Opelz G, Terasaki PI. Blood transfusions and kidney transplants: Remaining controversies. Transplant Proc 1981;13:136–41.
14. Buy-Quang D, Soulillou J.-P, Fontenaille Ch, Guimbretière J, Guenel J. Rôle bénéfique des transfusions sanguines et des grossesses dans la survie des allogreffes rénales. La Nouv Presse méd 1977;6,3503–7.
15. Persijn GG, Hooff JP van, Kalff MW, Lansbergen Q, Rood JJ van. Effect of blood transfusions and HLA matching on renal transplantation in the Netherlands. Transplant Proc 1977;9:503–5.
16. Bühlmann H, Largiadèr F, Uhlschmid G, Binswanger U, Binz H. Verlängertes Nierentransplantat – Uberleben dank Bluttransfusionen. Dtsch med

Wschr 1978;103:293–7.
17. Hourmant M, Soulillou JP, Buy-Quang D. Beneficial effect of blood transfusion. Transplantation 1979;28:40–3.
18. Oei LS, Thompson JS, Corry RJ. Effect of blood transfusions on survival of cadaver and living related renal transplants. Transplantation 1979; 28:482–4.
19. Betuel H, Touraine JL, Malik MC, Traeger J. Pretransplant protocols: Thoracic duct drainage, transfusions programmed and random, their effects on kidney graft survival. Transplant Proc 1981;13:167–71.
20. Opelz G, Terasaki PI. Prolongation effect of blood transfusion on kidney graft survival. Transplantation 1976;22:380–3.
21. Vincenti F, Duca RM, Amend W, et al. Immunologic factors determining survival of cadaver-kidney transplants. N Engl J Med 1978;299:793–8.
22. Alexandre GPJ, Cangh PJ van. Influence of blood transfusion on kidney transplantation. Dial Tranpl 1978;7:392–6.
23. Opelz G, Terasaki PI. International study of histocompatibility in renal transplantation. Transplantation 1982;33:87–95.
24. Opelz G, Graver B, Terasaki PI. Induction of high kidney graft survival rate by multiple transfusion. Lancet 1981;i:1223–5.
25. Opelz G, Terasaki PI. Importance of preoperative (not peroperative) transfusions for cadaver kidney transplants. Transplantation 1981;31: 106–8.
26. Caseley J, Moses VK, Lichter EA, Jonasson O. Isoimmunization of hemodialysis patients: Leukocyte-poor versus whole blood transfusions. Transplant Proc 1971;3:365–7.
27. Diepenhorst P, Sprokholt R, Prins HK. Removal of leukocytes from whole blood and erythrocyte suspensions by filtration through cotton wool. I. Filtration technique. Vox Sang 1972;23:308–20.
28. Persijn GG, Cohen B, Lansbergen Q, Rood JJ van. Retrospective and prospective studies on the effect of blood transfusions in renal transplantation in The Netherlands. Transplantation 1979;28:396–401.
29. Briggs JD, Canavan JSF, Dick HM, et al. Influence of HLA matching and blood transfusion on renal allograft survival. Transplantation 1978; 25:80–5.
30. Sirchia G. Blood transfusion and kidney transplantation. Dial Transpl 1978;7:390–1
31. Russell PS. Steps toward immediate progress in clinical transplantation. Transplant Proc 1977;9:1327–33.
32. Opelz G, Terasaki PI. Poor kidney-transplant survival in recipients with frozen-blood transfusions or no transfusions. Lancet 1974;ii: 696–8.
33. Säfwenberg J, Backman-Båve U, Högmann CF. The effect of blood transfusions on cadaver kidney transplants — an analysis of patients transplanted in Uppsala. Scand J Urol Nephrol (Suppl) 1977;42:59–61.
34. Polesky HF, McCullough JJ, Yunis E, et al. The effects of transfusion of frozen-thawed deglycerolized red cells on renal graft survival. Transplantation 1977;24:449–52.
35. Hunsicker LG, Oei LS, Freeman RM, Thomspon JS, Corry RJ. Effect of blood transfusions on cadaver renal allograft survival. Transplant Proc 1979;11:156–9.
36. Hamilton DNH, Watson MA, Briggs JD. Interrelation of pretransplant cell-mediated immunity, blood transfusion, and kidney transplant survival. Transplant Proc 1981;13:194–5.

37. Spees EK, Vaughn WK, Niblack G, et al. The effects of blood transfusion on cadaver renal transplantation: A prospective study of the Southeastern Organ Procurement Foundation 1977–1980. Transplant Proc 1981;13:155–160.
38. Fuller TC, Delmonico FL, Cosimi AB, Huggins CE, King M, Russell PS. Effects of various types of RBC transfusions on HLA alloimmunization and renal allograft survival. Transplant Proc 1977;9:117–9.
39. Blamey RW, Knapp MS, Burden RP, Salisbury M. Blood transfusion and renal allograft survival. Br Med J 1978;1:138–40.
40. Fehrman I, Ringdén O, Möller E, Lundgren G, Groth C.-G. Is cell-mediated immunity in the uremic patient affected by blood transfusion? Transplant Proc 1981;13:164–6.
41. Nubé MJ, Persijn GG, Kalff MW, Rood JJ van. Kidney transplantation – transplant survival after planned HLA-A and -B matched blood transfusions. Tissue Antigens 1981;17:449–54.
42. Albert ED, Scholz S, Meixner U, Land W. HLA-A, -B matching of pretransplant blood transfusion is associated with poor graft survival. Transplant Proc 1981;13:175–7.
43. Renterghem Y. van, Vandeputte I, Lerut T, Gruwez J, Vandeputte M, Michielsen P. HLA-A matched and HLA-B matched blood transfusions do not improve kidney allograft survival. New Engl J Med 1983;308:1102.
44. Borleffs JCC, Neuhaus P, Rood JJ van, Balner H. Platelet transfusions have a positive effect on kidney allograft survival in Rhesus monkeys without inducing cytotoxic antibodies. Lancet 1982;i:1117–8.
45. Werner-Favre C, Jeannet M, Harder F, Montadon A. Blood transfusions, cytotoxic antibodies, and kidney graft survival. Transplantation 1979;28:343–6.
46. Fauchet R, Wattelet J, Genetet B, Campion JP, Launois B, Cartier F. Role of blood transfusions and pregnancies in kidney transplantation. Vox Sang 1979;37:222–8.
47. Uldall PR, Wilkinson R, Dewar PJ, et al. Factors affecting the outcome of cadaver renal transplantation in Newcastle upon Tyne. Lancet 1977;ii:316–9.
48. Advisory Committee to the Renal Transplant Registry. The 13th report of the Human Renal Transplant Registry. Transplant Proc 1977;9:9–26.
49. Stiller CR, Lockwood BL, Sinclair NR, et al. Beneficial effect of operation-day blood-transfusions on human renal-allograft survival. Lancet 1978;i:169-70.
50. Brynger H, Frisk B, Sandberg L, Gelin L.-E. Renal graft rejection and blood transfusion before and during the transplant operation. Scand J Urol Nephrol 1978;12:271–3.
51. Persijn GG, Rood JJ van. Operation-day blood-transfusion and renal transplantation. Lancet 1978;i:495.
52. Solheim BG. The role of pretransplant blood transfusions. Transplant Proc 1979;11:138–44.
53. Fassbinder W, Frei U, Persijn G, et al. Graft survival in renal allograft recipients transfused perioperatively only. Transplant Proc 1982;14:164–7.
54. Glass NR, Felsheim G, Miller DT, Sollinger HW, Belzer FO. Influence of pre-and peri-operative blood transfusions on renal allograft survival. Transplantation 33, 1981;4:430–1.
55. Joysey VC, Roger JH, Evans DB, Herbertson BM. Differential kidney graft survival associated with interaction between recipient ABO group and

pretransplant blood transfusion. Transplantation 1977;24:371–6.
56. Bore PJ, Sells RA, Jamieson V, Burrows K. Transfusion-induced renal allograft protection. Transplant Proc 1979;11:148–51.
57. Opelz G, Terasaki PI. Effect of blood-group on relation between HLA match and outcome of cadaver kidney transplants. Lancet 1977;i:220–2.
58. Festenstein H, Bachoula-Papasteriadis C, Sachs JA, Jaraquemada D, Burke JM. Collaborative scheme for tissue typing and matching in renal transplantation. X. Effect of HLA-A, and B, D, and DR matching and pretransplant blood transfusion on 769 cadaver renal grafts. Transplant Proc 1979;11:752–5.
59. Fehrman I, Groth C-G, Lundgren G, Magnusson G, Möller E. Pretransplant dialysis and blood transfusion-correlation with cadaveric kidney graft survival. Transplant Proc 1979;11:152–5.
60. Guttmann RD. Interrelationship of time of dialysis-dependent uremia and pretransplant blood transfusions. Nephron 1978;22:196–200.
61. Andrus CH, Betts RF, May AG, Freeman RB. Cytomegalovirus infection blocks the beneficial effect of pretransplant blood transfusion on renal allograft survival. Transplantation 1979;28:451–6.
62. Tilikainen A, Kock B, Kuhlbäck B, Wallenius M. Transfusion and kidney graft survival in Finland. Scand J Urol Nephrol (Suppl) 1977;42:70–2.
63. Opelz G, Terasaki PI. Improvement of kidney-graft survival with increased numbers of blood transfusions. N Engl J Med 1978;299:799–803.
64. Ferrara GB, Tosi RM, Azzolina G, Carminati G, Longo A. HL-A unresponsiveness induced by weekly transfusions of small aliquots of whole blood. Transplantation 1974;17:194–200.
65. Zimmerman EC. Enhancing potential of whole blood. Transplant Proc 1977; 9:1081–5.
66. Ettinger RB, Terasaki I, Opelz G, et al. Successful renal allografts across a positive crossmatch for donor B-lymphocyte alloantigens. Lancet 1976;ii:56–8.
67. Iwaki Y, Terasaki PI, Park MS, Billing R. Enhancement of human kidney allografts by cold B-lymphocyte cytotoxins. Lancet 1978;i:1228–9.
68. Jeannet M, Vassali P, Hufschmid MF. Enhancement of human kidney allografts by cold B lymphocyte cytotoxins. Transplantation 1980;29:174–7.
69. Suciu-Foca N, Rohowsky C, Kung P, et al. MHC specific idiotypes on alloactivated human T cells. In vivo and in vitro studies. Transplant Proc 1983;15:784–9.
70. Singal DP, Joseph S, Szewcuk MR. Possible mechanism of the beneficial effect of pretransplant blood transfusions on renal allograft survival in man. Transplant Proc 1983;14:316–8.
71. Rood JJ van, Balner H. Blood transfusion and transplantation. Transplantation 1978;26:275.
72. Smith MD, Williams JD, Coles GA, Salaman JR. The effect of blood transfusion on T-suppressor cells in renal dialysis patients. Transplant Proc 1981;13:181–3.
73. Fisher E, Lenhard V, Seifert P, Kluge A, Johannsen R. Blood transfusion induced suppression of cellular immunity in man. Hum Immunol 1980;3: 187–94.
74. Keown PA, Descamps B. Improved renal allograft survival after blood transfusion: a non-specific, erythrocyte mediated immunoregulatory process? Lancet 1979;i:20–2.
75. Goulmy E, Persijn GG, Blokland EC, D'Amaro J, Rood JJ van. Cell-mediated lympholysis studies in renal allograft recipients. Transplantation 1981;31:210–7.

ROLE OF LYMPHOCYTES IN GRAFT-VERSUS-HOST DISEASE AND ITS PREVENTION

D.W. van Bekkum

INTRODUCTION

The most frequent complication to occur after the take of an incompatible bone marrow graft is graft-versus-host disease (GvHD) in any of its various forms. It is now commonly accepted that this disease is caused by an immunological reaction of T lymphocytes which have been transferred with the graft itself or by T lymphocytes which develop from grafted precursor cells. The GvH reaction is directed against the tissue antigens of the recipient leading to pathological changes in many organs: the skin, the intestinal tract and the liver being most frequently and severely affected. In general, GvHD develops only following transplantation of allogeneic or xenogeneic bone marrow, but a similar syndrome has been observed occasionally when syngeneic bone marrow is grafted under very special conditions. In all animal species studied so far, the symptomatology of GvDH proved to be very similar. Most of the information available today is derived from mice, rats, dogs and monkeys and of course from the human transplant patients.

PATTERNS OF GVHD AND MORTALITY

The severity and the course of secondary disease vary among different species and also within a species, depending on the source, nature and number of the grafted cells. The most severe form following MHC mismatched allogeneic bone marrow transplantation has been encountered in Rhesus monkeys (1) and the limited experience with human patients has suggested a similarly severe course (2). Mortality in the Rhesus monkey may occur so early (mean survival time 13 days) that it falls within the period in which death from bone marrow failure occurs in untreated controls. The two causes of death can only be differentiated accurately by microscopic examination of the affected tissues.

Following transplantation of allogeneic or xenogeneic bone marrow, irradiated mice rapidly recover from radiation sickness and begin to gain weight during the second week. However, between 20 and 30 days after the transplantation the faeces become moisty and the animals start to lose weight again, which may give rise to varying degrees of wasting. In a proportion of the animals characteristic skin lesions appear as early as the beginning of the second month. These lesions may either subside, or persist for many months. In mice transplanted with allogeneic bone marrow, the peak of mortality from GvLH is in the second and third month, thereafter the symptoms subside and mortality decreases (Fig. 1). When the genetic difference

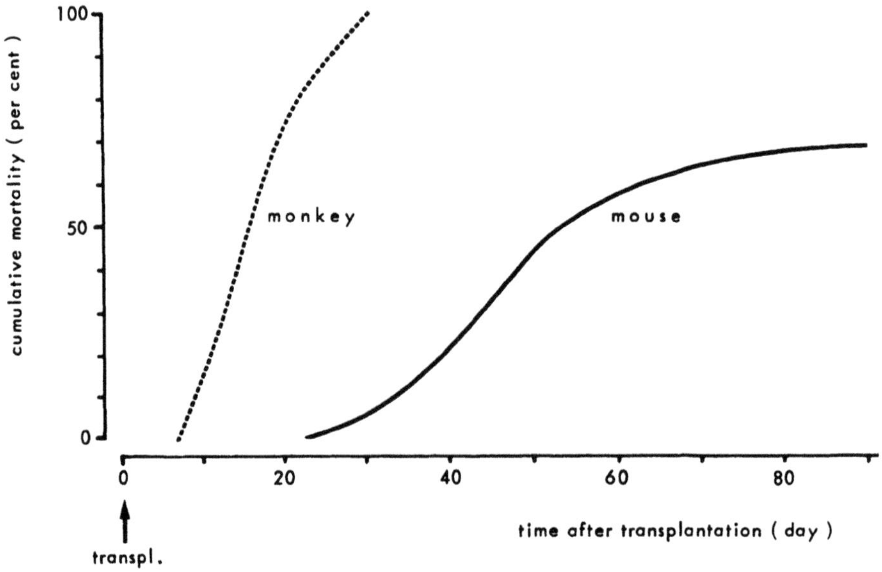

Figure 1. Patterns of mortality from GvHD in Rhesus monkeys and mice grafted with MHC incompatible bone marrow cells after a lethal dose of total body irradiation.

between host and donor is relatively large, e.g. in the case of rat → mouse chimeras, the recovery after the third month may be less obvious, but a certain decrease in the severity of the symptoms is nearly always apparent. The course of GvHD in allogeneic rat chimeras resembles that seen in mice, except that skin lesions and wasting were more prominent in rats (3). In the surviving rats the lesions had a tendency to disappear at the end of the third month and almost complete recovery occurred in the majority of the animals. Recently, Beschorner (4) described a chronic type of GvHD in rats developing in long-term allogeneic chimeras between 6 and 12 months after transplantation in about 50% of the animals which survive the acute GvHD.

A similarly rapid and fatal course of GvHD as is seen in monkeys grafted with MHC mismatched allogeneic bone marrow (1) can be induced in mice by the injection of allogeneic lymphoid cells in addition to allogeneic bone marrow. The animals may die as early as the 6th day following transplantation without having developed a clearly defined clinical syndrome. This kind of death can be distinguished, nevertheless, from early radiation death on the basis of histological changes. With lower numbers of lymph node or spleen cells added to the bone marrow graft, the resulting GvHD in mice is subacute and mortality occurs later, the lower the number of lymphocytes grafted (5).

In the dog, long-term uncomplicated survival is the rule following a graft of DLA identical bone marrow from a sibling donor. Occasionally, GvH reactions of the delayed type occur, but these are usually transient and fatal GvHD occurs in less than 5% of the grafted animals. The absence of acute

GvHD in such donor-recipient combinations can be explained by the low concentration of post-thymic T cells in dog bone marrow. When donor lymph node cells are added to the DLA matched bone marrow graft, the severity and incidence of GvHD accordingly increases (6). Following a take of DLA mismatched marrow from an unrelated donor, dogs develop actue GvHD which is usually fatal within one month.

Thus, broadly one can distinguish an acute type of GvHD which starts within one to two weeks after grafting and a delayed type which begins about one month or even later after transplantation. The acute form occurs only when a sufficiently large number of lymphoid cells are present among the grafted cells and it has to be ascribed to the reactivity of the grafted lymphocytes and their descendants. Proliferation of clones of these grafted lymphocytes probably occurs as a result of continuous antigenic stimulation by the tissue antigens of the recipient. Removal of these cells from the graft or their inactivation prior to transplantation precludes the development of this form of GvHD. The acute GvH reaction is not dependent on the presence of a thymus gland, since it proceeds unchanged in thymectomized recipients. In contrast, the delayed type of GvHD, which characteristically occurs following grafting of moderate numbers of allogeneic H-2 different mouse bone marrow cells, can be prevented by thymectomy of the recipients (7). Delayed type GvHD is therefore attributed to post-thymic T lymphocytes which are generated from prethymic precursor cells under the influence of the thymic microenvironment. In the case of a small antigenic difference between donor and recipient, e.g. MHC identity, these cells may acquire a state of immunological tolerance towards the recipient. The two mechanisms, thymus-independent and thymus-dependent, are very difficult to unravel by clinical observations only, since small numbers of grafted post-thymus T lymphocytes can produce a late form of GvHD which is indistinguishable from the thymus-dependent type (Fig. 2) (5).

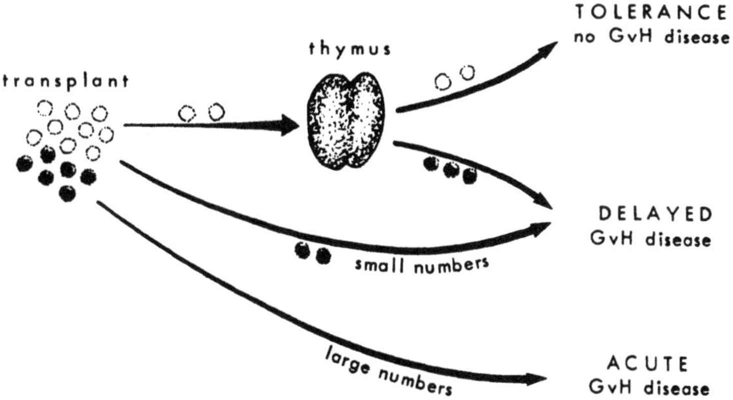

Figure 2. Postulated mechanism of development of acute delayed type GvHD. Acute type: by preformed post-thymic T lymphocytes which initiate reactive clones. Large numbers of lymphocytes required. Occurs with MHC mismatched and matched donors. Delayed type: by prethymic precursors which mature in the thymus. MHC mismatch; or by small numbers of post-thymic MHC mismatched T lymphocytes; or by larger numbers of post-thymic MHC identical T lymphocytes.

In patients grafted before the area of tissue typing (2) acute and fatal GvHD occurred in the majority of cases. Acute GvHD is a frequent and mostly fatal complication of transfusion of (unirradiated) blood in SCID patients and has also occurred, but less frequently, in adult patients who received large amounts of granulocyte transfusions as supportive treatment for leukemia and Hodgkin's disease (8–10).

Bone marrow grafting with HLA identical siblings as donors results in clinical GvHD in an average of 50% of the cases, depending on the characteristics of the patient group and the centre. The disease may develop early with all the characteristics of acute GvHD or as late as 3 months after grafting. The disease once established runs a fatal course in about half of the cases. In addition, a chronic debilitating form of GvHD is seen following allogeneic marrow transplantation, which is characterized by Lichen planus, scleroderma-like skin lesions, a Sicca syndrome including the eyes, the mouth, the oesophagus and the vaginal vault; serosal involvement, infections and immune function abnormalities, which may persist for years (11–14). In one centre, this chronic cutaneous GvHD, as it has been termed, was observed in 30% of patients who survived beyond 150 days after transplantation.

THE ROLE OF T LYMPHOCYTES IN THE DEVELOPMENT OF GVHD

Bone marrow contains immunocompetent T lymphocytes and their proportion varies in different species (table I). Accordingly, increasing the number of bone marrow cells grafted increases the risk of development of GvHD, provided there are immunogenetic differences between donor and recipient.

Table I. GvHD and T lymphocytes in bone marrow of different species.

	Mouse	Dog	Monkey	Human
Graft versus host disease				
allo MHC match		50% (mild)	100% (mild) severe)	50% (mild/
MHC mismatch	delayed	acute severe	acute severe	acute
T lymphocytes in BM	few	intermediate	many	many

In patients, bone marrow is most frequently employed for the treatment of aplasia and leukemia, but fetal liver cells as well as blood nucleated cells have been proposed. For the treatment of patients, all these tissues as well as thymus cell suspensions have actually been employed. In experimental animals, spleen and lymph node suspensions have been studied extensively as well. The cellular composition of these various tissues differ between different species and with age.

When compared in the same GvH assay, lymph node cells are most potent, followed by spleen cells, adult thymus, bone marrow and fetal liver. Peripheral blood cells are compared to spleen cells. Spleen cells from athymic nude mice can elicit a delayed-type of GvHD, but do not enhance GvH when added to a normal allogeneic bone marrow graft (15). Fetal thymus in the mouse has negligible GvH inducing potential. All hemopoietic tissues which contain sufficient stem cells to produce a take, seem to have the capacity of inducing delayed-type GvHD when donor and recipient are MHC mismatched. Even with fetal liver delayed type GvHD occurs in mice, be it with less frequency than following bone marrow transplantation. The difference between fetal liver and bone marrow cannot be fully explained by the difference in the proportion of mature T cells, since the same difference was still found when bone marrow or fetal liver cells were depleted of T lymphocytes by discontinuous gradient centrifugation (16). In monkeys and man the bone marrow contains abundant T cells. In these species MHC mismatched grafts induce acute GvHD, of a severity that is only seen in mice with spleen or lymph node cell grafts. With MHC matched donor marrow, GvHD develops in about 50% of the human patients and in all Rhesus monkeys. Most cases are of the delayed type, but acute GvHD under these conditions is by no means infrequent. In the dog, MHC matched donor marrow causes only very mild GvHD of the delayed type and mortality from this cause is rare. In mice, a large excess of H-2 identical marrow is needed to cause some acute GvHD. This indicates that the proportion of T cells in dog marrow is intermediate between that of the mouse and the primates. The number of T lymphocytes in peripheral blood of human is such that blood transfusions can be a real hazard for immune paralyzed patients (table II) (17). There are a series of reports in the literature of SCID patients who developed fatal GvHD following a transfusion of a relatively small amount of blood (18). Some cases of GvHD have also been reported in immunocompromised removal adults who were given large amounts of granulocyte rich blood.

Table II. Induction of GvHD by blood transfusions.

- 1 l blood contains 18 x 10^8 lymphocytes.
- 1.5 x 10^7 mouse spleen cells/kg → 50% GvHD in immune suppressed recipient mice.
- This number is equivalent to 600 ml of blood for an adult immuno-paralyzed patient.
- 7/33 patients* receiving ∿ 1 l of blood from CML donors (6 x 10^7 ly/kg) developed GvHD (17).
- 30 ml of fresh blood may cause GvHD in a baby with SCID.
- GvH inducing capacity is diminished but not destroyed by cryopreservation, storage at 4°C and by incubation for 1 h at 37°C.

* Agranulocytic leukemic patients having received high dose chemotherapy.

PREVENTION OF GVHD

For preventing GvHD induced by transfusions of blood or blood products it is most practical to irradiate the transfusion before infusion. The products or cells of interest in transfusions (erythrocytes, granulocytes, platelets) are not functionally impaired by the radiation doses needed to inactivate lymphocytes. The dose of X- or γ-radiation required for abrogating the

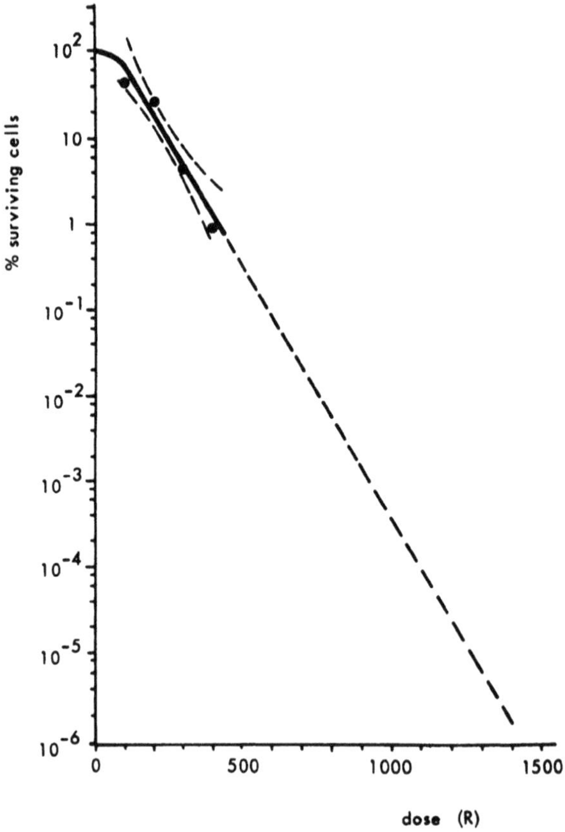

Figure 3. Survival curve of mouse lymph node cells following in vitro irradiation. The curve is extrapolated from the data published by Smith and Vos (19). The extrapolated portion is represented by the broken part of the line. In the report the dose of radiation is measured in R; for practical purposes the abcissa may be read in current rad units.

risk of induction of GvHD from 500 ml of blood or the equivalent number of lymphocytes (7–15 x 10^8) contained in blood products, is derived from the dose-survival curve depicted in figure 3 (19). A dose of 1500 rad will reduce the viable lymphocytes in 500 ml of fresh blood to 7–15 when the cells are irradiated under conditions of full oxygenation. When the irradiated blood is anoxic the dose required to achieve the same effect is 3 times as high. When the oxygenation of the blood cannot be specifically controlled, as will probably be the case in clinical practice, it is recommended that the dose of irradiation be doubled to 3000 rads, which is in accordance with recommendations by Coifman et al. (20,21). Blood stored for a limited period of time should be irradiated before it is administered to such patients. In most centres 2000 rad is delivered to transfusion bags. Under anoxic conditions this would result in a reduction of viable lymphocytes by a factor of 10^3–10^4 which is probably also sufficient. There is no recorded case of thus irradiated blood or blood products having caused GvHD in a patient.

While radical inactivation of lymphocytes can be easily carried out in blood by irradiation, this treatment cannot be employed for the same purpose in bone marrow transplants because radiation will similarly inactivate the pluripotent hemopoietic stem cells that are essential for rescuing the recipient.

A variety of methods has been explored to selectively remove or inactivate T lymphocytes in bone marrow in vitro, among these are separations by density gradient centrifugation, by lectin adherence or adherence to sheep erythrocytes, inactivation with anti-lymphocytic polyclonal antibodies or monoclonal antibodies.

All of these technques have been developed in animal models and are presently being tested for their efficacy in the clinical situation.

Another, most effective method to mitigate GvHD is bacteriological decontamination and reverse barrier nursing of the recipient. Treatment with ALG, corticosteroids or cyclosporin A after the transplantation also has a significant abrogating effect of variable magnitude in individual patients. One problem which complicates the removal or inactivation of T lymphocytes from allogeneic bone marrow grafts is the finding that this depletion reduces the rate of regeneration of hemopoiesis or may even prevent to neutralize that effect, but such measures also increase the toxicity of the conditioning procedure. Therefore a combination of T lymphocyte depletion with post transplantation treatment with ALG or cyclosporin A seems to be the best approach.

It will take some years before the results of these clinical studies will be available.

REFERENCES

1. De Vries MJ, Crouch BG, Van Putten LM, Van Bekkum DW. Pathological changes in irradiated monkeys treated with bone marrow. J Nat Cancer Inst 1961;27:67–97.
2. Mathé G, Bernard J, De Vries MJ, et al. Nouveaux essais de greffe de moëlle osseuse homologue après irradiation totale chez des enfants atteints de leucémie aiguë en rémission. Rev Hémat 1960;15:115–61.
3. Balner H, De Vries MJ, Van Bekkum DW. Secondary disease in rat radiation chimeras. J Nat Cancer Inst 1964;32:419–59.
4. Beschorner WE, Tutschka PJ, Santos GW. Chronic graft-versus-host disease in the rat radiation chimera. Transplantation 1982;33:393–9.
5. Heidt PJ, Wagemaker G, Knaan-Shanzer S, Van Bekkum DW. Two distinct types of late onset graft-versus-host disease after bone marrow transplantation in lethally irradiated mice. Transplantation 1981;32:263–4.
6. Vriesendorp HM, Bijnen AB, Van Kessel ACM, Obertop H, Westbroek DL. Minor histocompatibility systems in dogs. In: Baum SJ, Ledney GD, eds. Experimental hematology today 1978. New York, Springer Verlag: 1978: 109–17.
7. Van Putten LM. Thymectomy: Effect on secondary disease in radiation chimeras. Science 1964;145:935–6.

8. Weiden PL, Zuckerman N, Hansen JA, et al. Fatal graft-versus-host disease in patient with lymphoblastic leukemia following normal granulocyte transfusion. Blood 1981;57:328–32.
9. Van Bekkum DW. Transfusion or transplantation? Isr J Med Sci 1965;1:870–82.
10. Dinsmore RE, Straus DJ, Pollack MS, et al. Fatal graft-versus-host disease following blood transfusion in Hodgkin's disease documented by HLA typing. Blood 1980;55:831–4.
11. Graze PR, Gale RP. Chronic graft-versus-host disease: a syndrome of disordered immunity. Am J Med 1979;66:611–20.
12. Sullivan KM, Shulman HM, Storb R, et al. Chronic graft-versus-host disease in 52 patients; adverse natural course and successful treatment with combination immunosuppression. Blood 1981;57:267–76.
13. Shulman HM, Sale GE, Lerner KG, et al. Chronic cutaneous graft-versus-host disease in man. Am J Path 1978;91:545–70.
14. Shulman HM, Sullivan KM, Weiden PL, et al. Chronic graft-versus-host syndrome in man: A clinopathological study of 20 long-term Seattle patients. Am J Med 1980;69:204–17.
15. O'Kunewick JP, Meredith RF, Raikov RB, Brozovich BJ, Magliere K. Fatal response suggestive of graft-versus-host reaction following transplantation of spleen cells from allogeneic athymic (nude) donors. Transplantation 1981;31:201–4.
16. Löwenberg B, De Zeeuw MHC, Dicke KA, Van Bekkum DW. Nature of the graft-versus-host reactivity of fetal liver cell transplants in mice. J Nat Cancer Inst 1977;58:959–66.
17. Schwarzenberg L, Mathé G, De Grouchy J, et al. White blood cell transfusions. Isr J Med Sci 1965;1:925–56.
18. Van Bekkum DW. Use and abuse of hemopoietic cell grafts in immune deficiency diseases. Transplant Rev 1972;9:3–53.
19. Smith LH, Vos O. Radiation sensitivity of mouse lymph node cells relative to their proliferative capacity in vivo. Radiat Res 1963;19:485–91.
20. Coifman RE, Meuwissen HJ. Elimination of graft-versus-host competent lymphocytes from transfusable blood components by radiation. Fed Proc 1971;30:456.
21. Coifman RE, Good RA, Meuwissen HJ. The function of irradiated blood elements. I. Limitations on the response to phytohemagglutinin as an indicator of immunocompetence in irradiated lymphocytes. Proc Soc Exp Biol NY 1971;137:155–60.

SELECTIVE DECONTAMINATION OF THE DIGESTIVE TRACT AS A METHOD OF INFECTION PREVENTION IN GRANULOCYTOPENIC PATIENTS; A FOLLOW-UP STUDY IN 102 PATIENTS

H.G. de Vries-Hospers, D.Th. Sleijfer, N.H. Mulder, H.O. Nieweg and D. van der Waaij

INTRODUCTION

Several years ago selected decontamination of the digestive tract (SDD) (1) was proposed for prevention of infection in the neutropenic patient. This method aims at elimination of potentially pathogenic bacteria from the gut without affecting the anaerobic microflora. From the infection preventing point of view this is acceptable because anaerobic bacteria seldomly cause infections in the granulocytopenic patient (2). On the other hand anaerobes have been shown to play a key role in the normal interbacterial balance. The presence of an intact anaerobic flora in the gut hinders colonization by potentially pathogenic bacteria such as aerobic Gram-negative bacilli, yeasts and staphylococci. The mechanism which prevents colonization by potentially pathogenic microorganisms (ppmo) in the gut has been first described by Van der Waaij who introduced the term colonization resistance (CR) (3). The above mentioned ppmo are also the most frequently involved ppmo in infections in the neutropenic patient (2). The majority of these infections find their porte of entry in the digestive tract (4). In order to prevent infection it is therefore attempted to clear the digestive tract from these potentially pathogenic microorganisms. Moreover it was attempted to preserve an intact CR, so that the natural barrier against colonization is at least maintained. It may even be artificially increased by oral administration of antimicrobial agents which are able to eliminate selectively certain ppmo. In a prospective controlled clinical trial SDD appeared to be effective in reducing the infection frequency (1). The difference however was only significant at granulocyte levels below $0.5x10^9/l$.

SDD is now applied routinely to patients with hematological malignancies and less than $0.5x10^9/l$ granulocytes. In this follow-up study the results of SDD in 102 granulocytopenic patients are presented. In order to be able to compare these results with those obtained in the previous study (1), the latter patients were re-evaluated only for those period they experienced granulocyte counts below $0.1x10^9/l$ for at least one week.

PATIENTS AND METHODS

Patients

Adult patients with acute myeloid (AML) or acute lymphoid leukemia (ALL) in whom aggressive chemotherapy resulting in severe neutropenia was considered as well as patients with aplastic anemia who had less than $0.5x10^9$ granulocytes per l of blood were entered in the study. Patients with acute lymphoid leukemia were treated with a regimen which consisted of vincristine, prednisone and l-asparaginase. Daunorubicin was added when indicated. Acute myeloid leukemia was treated with a regimen consisting of arabinosyl cytosine, 6-thioguanine and daunorubicin (5). Second remission inductions were performed with the same regimen with a higher dose of arabinosyl cytosine (650 mg/m^2).

1. Aerobic Gram-negative bacilli. Enterobacteriaceae-species were eliminated with either nalidixic acid (8 g/day) or co-trimoxazole (2880 mg/day) or polymyxin B or E (800 mg/day). Proteus-species are essentially resistant to the latter drug. Pseudomonas-species were eliminated by polymyxin.
2. Yeasts and fungi. Both amphotericin B (1-2 g/day) and nystatin (6.10^6 I.U./day) are suitable for this purpose. Amphotericin B has preference because most of the yeasts are more susceptible to this drug.
3. S. aureus can effectively be eliminated by oral administration of cefradin in a daily dose of 6 grams.

All drugs were given orally and as long as the patients were granulocytopenic. Drugs from group 1 and 2 were given to all patients. Which one of the drugs was used for elimination of Gram-negative bacilli was left to the judgement of the clinician. However patient factors such as allergy or kidney function disturbance as well as the sensitivity pattern of the isolated microorganisms were taken in consideration. Usually one of the drugs was given at the time. Cefradin was added only on indication i.e. colonization by S. aureus. The antimycotic drugs were preferably given as a suspension. The other antimicrobial agents were given as tablets.

Microbiological surveillance

Before the SDD-drugs were administered inventory cultures from the faeces and the throat swabs were performed. Thereafter these cultures were performed three times a week as long as SDD was continued. The cultures were performed only aerobically. A one gram fecal sample was diluted 1:10 in brain heart infusion (BHI) broth (Oxoid) and incubated overnight at 37°C. Thereafter subinoculations were made on MacConkey (MC) agar (Oxoid) as well as on yeast morphology (YM) agar (Merck) in order to be able to quantitate Gram-negative bacilli and yeasts respectively. All macroscopically different colonies of Gram-negative bacilli on the MC agar were identified according to the API-system (6). Sensitivity patterns were determined from all different API-types. This was done for all SDD-drugs as well as for a number of drugs currently in use for the systemic therapy in the case of a suspected infection.

Hematological surveilance

White blood cell counts were counted in the Coulter counter ($> 3x10^9$ cells/l) or in a counting chamber ($< 3x10^9$ cells /l). Absolute levels of granulocytes were counted in the hemocytometer or calculated from a differential count of the total white blood cell count. Differential counting was performed on 300 cells in a buffy coat smear. Counting of granulocytes was performed three times a week.

Clinical surveillance and treatment

Complete physical and radiographic examination of the chest and the sinuses as well as microbiological investigations were performed in each patient on the first day on study and repeated when the patient had fever. In case of a suspected infection, other specimens i.e. blood, urine, sputum or pus were cultured. When axillary temperature rose above 38.5°C blood cultures were taken. All patients were treated in conventional ward rooms of four beds under standard conditions. Non-sterile food and beverages were supplied. Patients who lost more than 10% of their body weight were fed by intragastric tube in addition (7). For this purpose we used sterile tube feeding during the last half year of the study.

When indicated supportive treatment was given including red blood cells, granulocytes or platelet transfusions as well as broad spectrum bactericidal antibiotics (gentamicin, tobramycin, cefradin, cefuroxime, ticarcillin) and local or systemic antifungal therapy (amphotericin B plus 5-fluorocytosine). Local antimycotic therapy consisted of oral application of amphotericin B in Orabase® (8) or as lozenges, each containing 10 mg of amphotericin B (9).

Registration of acquired infections

Fever was defined as axillary temperature above 38.5°C. A microbiologically documented infection was defined as the presence of definite signs and symptoms of an infection plus the isolation and identification of ppmo from blood, urine, sputum or local sites. A clinical documented infection was defined as the presence of definite signs and symptoms of infection with negative cultures. Infection days were defined as days on which the patient had fever due to clinically or microbiologically documented infections.

Non-infectious allergic fever was fever associated with a non-infectious cause like blood transfusion, administration of antileukemic or antimicrobial therapy. Fever of unknown origin was defined as fever not associated with signs or symptoms of infections and without positive cultures or manifest allergic reactions. An infectious episode was a period during which the patient had fever due to a clinically or microbiologically documented infection.

RESULTS

Patients

Of the 102 patients, 17 had aplastic anemia, 28 had ALL and 57 had AML. The patients were studied during 3008 days in total resulting in an average study time per patient of 29.4 days. During 60% of this period the granulocyte count was less than $0.1x10^9$/l (Table I).

Acquired infections

In total 30 severe acquired infection were registered. Microbiological documentation was obtained for 16 infectious episodes. All infections except one occurred during the period the patient experienced less than $0.1x10^9$ granulocytes/l. Microbiological documentation was obtained for 16 infections. Localisation and causative microorganisms of the infections are listed in Table II.

Table I. Number of study days in 102 neutropenic patients.

Diagnosis	Number of patients	Number of days with granulocyte counts $x10^9/l$		
		0.1–5	< 0.1	< 0.5
AML	57	560	1321	1881
ALL	28	397	372	769
AA	17	200	158	358
All diagnosis	102	1157	1851	3008

AML = acute myeloid leukemia.
ALL = acute lymphoid leukemia.
AA = aplastic anemia.

Table II. Localisation and causative microorganisms of 30 severe acquired infections in 102 SDD patients with < $0.5x10^9$ granulocytes/l.

Causative micro-organism	Septicemia	Pulmonary infections	Infections of skin and soft tissue	Meningeal infections	Oropharyngeal area
P. aeruginosa	3	-	1	-	1
C. albicans	1	1	-	-	-
Aspergillus	-	1	-	-	-
S. epidermidis	3	-	-	-	-
Enterococci	2	-	-	-	-
B. cereus	1	-	-	-	-
Diptheroid rods	-	-	-	1	-
Clinical infections	-	8	3	-	4
All infections	10	10	4	1	5

The number of both microbiologically and clinically documented infectious episodes per 100 patient days during which the patients experienced granulocyte counts below $0.1x10^9/l$ was 1.5. During the re-evaluated trial period this figure was 1.4 (Table III).

Days with infection as percentage of days on study were 6.8 for the whole group and 11.4 for the patient with less than 11.4 for the pateints with less than $0.1x10^9$ granulocytes/l.

During 2244 study days the patients received only one of the drugs available for selective elimination of Gram-negative bacilli. Combinations were given on the other days. Days with infection as percentage of the days on study with one of the SDD-drugs were 5.3 for nalidixic acid, 6.8 for co-trimoxazole and 11.2 for polymyxin.

Table III. SDD patients with < $0.5x10^9$ granulocytes/l: infections during the period the granulocyte count was < $0.1x10^9$/l.

	Trial period	Post-trial period
Number of patients studied	41	102
Number of study days	1026	3008
Number of days with granulocytes < $0.1x10^9$/l	505/1026=49.2%	1851/3008=61.5%
Number of days with granulocytes <$0.1x10^9$/l per patient	505/41=12.3%	1851/102=18.1%
Number of severe acquired infections (clinically + microbiologically documented)	7	29
Number of severe acquired infections per patient	0.2	0.3
Number of severe acquired infections per 100 patient days with granulocyte count < $0.1x10^9$/l	1.4	1.5

Microbiological surveillance

Inventory. In all 102 cases Gram-negative bacilli were found in the inventory cultures of the feces, in 26 cases these microorganisms were also cultured from the throat swabs. The Gram-negative bacilli isolated from these cultures were sensitive to nalidixic acid in 98%, to co-trimoxazole in 95% and to polymyxin in 80%. In no cases microorganisms were resistant to all three antimicrobial agents. Yeasts were cultured from 20% of the fecal cultures and from 57% of the throat swabs.

Selective decontamination. In all patients the feces were free of the target Gram-negative bacilli within one week after starting SDD; in the patients initially treated with polymixin this effect was obtained even sooner, namely in one or two days. However, when *Proteus*-species were isolated from the inventory flora, these bacteria only disappeared after the administration of either nalidixic acid or co-trimoxazole.

After the fecal cultures had become free of Gram-negative bacilli, this situation could be maintained during the whole SDD-period in 43 patients. Gram-negative bacilli were cultured only once in 25 patients and two or more times in 34. Of the Gram-negative bacilli isolated during SDD 73% was sensitive to the drugs used for SDD on the moment of occurrence of the positive fecal culture. For 60% of the resistant bacteria readjustment of treatment was necessary because the concentration of the resistant bacterium rose or the culture did not become negative without a change in the SDD-regimen.

As mentioned above, resistance to the SDD-drugs occurred. However, only in 8 cases it could be made likely that resistance had been developed as the same API-type was isolated previously while it was still sensitive.

This was observed three times in patients treated with nalidixic acid and five times in co-trimoxazole-treated patients. During treatment with polymixin this was never seen. Moreover this occurred only during the first week after initiation of SDD.

DISCUSSION

In this follow-up study concerning 102 neutropenic SDD-patients 30 severe acquired infections were registered. The majority of these infections (29/30=97%) occurred during the period the patients had less than $0.1x10^9$ granulocytes/l. Microbiological documentation was found for 16 out of these 30 infections. Of the causative microorganisms 8 belonged to the group of Gram-negative bacilli and yeasts (Table II), against which SDD was directed. The *Pseudomonas*-septicemia's were preceded by gastrointestinal colonization. All these patients received tube feeding via a nasogastric tube. Later on it appeared that the tube feeding was contaminated by *Pseudomonas*-species. After the institution of sterile tube feeding such food-borne outbreaks of *Pseudomonas*-septicemia's were no longer seen.

The average number of severe acquired infections per patient was 0.3 (Table III). As the mean study time per patient amounted 2.4 days the mean number of infectious episodes per 100 patient days can be calculated and is about 1. For the period the patients had less than $0.1x10^9$ granulocytes/l this figure was 1.5 (Table III). This figure did not differ from that obtained during the re-evaluated trial period – where it was 1.4 – although the patients during the follow-up study were at risk for a longer period.

The percentages of fever days during treatment with one of the absorbable drugs alone was lower (5.3% and 6.8% respectively) than during treatment with the nonabsorbable polymyxin (11.2%). Although this study was not performed to investigate the effect on infection prevention of either drug alone, retrospective evaluation of these data suggests at least an additional systemic effect of the absorbable SDD-drugs. Recently Wade et al. (10) published the results of a study in which nalidixic acid was compared with co-trimoxazole; the latter drug appeared to be superior for prevention of infections. Also Kurrle et al. (11) demonstrated that an SDD-regimen in which co-trimoxazole was included was superior to a fixed combination of polymyxin, neomycin and low dose nalidixic acid as it is used by the Leiden group (12,13). However, as yet no studies have been performed in which polymyxin alone was compared with one of the absorbable drugs alone.

Elimination of fecal Gram-negative bacilli cultured from the inventory flora was in general no problem. This situation could be maintained in 43% of the patients during the whole granulocytopenic period which lasted on the average 29.4 days. In the other patients one or more positive fecal cultures were found during the SDD-period. The majority of these Gram-negative bacilli however was susceptible to the drugs used for SDD on the moment of occurrence of the positive culture. The susceptible bacteria disappeared without adjustment of the SDD-regimen. This applied also for 40% of the resistant bacteria. This is in accordance with earlier experience of our group (14) which also showed that contaminations not always resulted in colonizations. Although this is difficult to substantiate, we believe that an intact CR may have contributed to this phenomenon. However, when contamination was followed by colonization the treatment was adjusted according to the sensitivity pattern of the isolated Gram-negative bacilli which promptly resulted in negative fecal cultures.

The development of resistance was seen in 8 cases. This occurred only during the first week after the start of SDD and only in those patients who were initially treated with the absorbable nalidixic acid or co-trimoxazole. The explanation may be found in the fact that it took about one week before the cultures could be expected to be negative after initiation of these drugs. During this period the fecal concentration of these drugs will gradually increase until a steady state has been reached after about a week. The effect of oral administration of polymyxin was reflected in the feces within a few days. This rapid disappearance of Gram-negative bacilli seems to be important in the prevention of development of resistance. For that reason we advocate to start SDD with a drug which is able to eliminate susceptible Gram-negative bacilli as soon as possible. Polymyxin is the most suitable drug for this purpose. If the results of the inventory cultures are not yet available at the beginning of SDD a second drug is added. The same is done when the inventory flora is not fully sensitive to polymyxin alone. Later on when the surveillance cultures are free of Gram-negative bacilli, SDD is performed with one of the drugs at a time. This is done both for economic reasons as well as to reduce the number of tablets to be swallowed by the patient. Maintenance of SDD with one of the drugs at a time increases however the chance for the finding of positive surveillance cultures as the spectrum of ppmo covered is smaller. Patients are treated in the open ward and receive non-sterilized hospital food. Therefore they are exposed daily to environmental bacteria which may contaminate the patient. To compensate for the disadvantage of maintenance of SDD with one single drug surveillance cultures were performed thrice weekly. In this way we were able to intervene rather rapidly when feces- or throat-swab cultures indicated so. Adequate readjustment of the SDD-regimen can prevent the increase in resistant strains. This can also be reduced by using a fixed combination of polymyxin and co-trimoxazole (15).

The compliance of the SDD-regimen by the patient was not measured in this study. However, the oral intake of the drugs was sufficient to eliminate susceptible Gram-negative bacilli within a reasonable period of time (one week).

In comparison with total decontamination SDD is more convenient to the patient. Moreover the costs are lower as there is no absolute need for strict reverse isolation. However, as the patients are continuously exposed to environmental sources of ppmo such as food and the hands of the medical staff, frequent microbiological monitoring is necessary and the finding of positive cultures must result in readjustment of the SDD-regimen.

REFERENCES

1. Sleijfer DT, Mulder NH, De Vries-Hospers HG, et al. Infection prevention in granulocytopenic patients by selective decontamination of the digestive tract. Eur J Cancer 1980;16:859–69.
2. Bodey GP, Rodriguez V, Chang HY, Narboni G. Fever and infection in leukemic patients. Cancer 1978;41:1610–22.
3. Van der Waaij D, Berghuis-de Vries JM, Lekkerkerk-van der Wees JEC. Colonization resistance of the digestive tract in conventional and antibiotic treated animals. J Hyg Camb 1971;69:405–11.

4. Schimpff SC, Young VM, Greene WH, Vermeulen GD, Moody MR, Wiernik PH. Origin of infection in acute nonlymphocytic leukemia. Significance of hospital acquired infections. Ann Intern Med 1972;77:707–14.
5. Gale RP, Cline MJ. High remission induction rate in acute myeloid leukemia. Lancet 1977;i:497–9.
6. Smith PB, Tomforde KM, Rhoden DL, Balows A. API-system: A multitube method for indentification of Enterobacteriaceae. Appl Microbiol 1972; 24:449–52.
7. De Vries EGE, Mulder NH, Houwen BH, De Vries-Hospers HG. Enteral nutrition by nasogastric tube in adult patients treated with intensive chemotherapy for acute leukemia. Am J Clin Nutrition 1982;35:1490–6.
8. De Vries-Hospers HG, Van der Waaij D. Amphotericin B concentrations in saliva after application of 2% amphotericin B in Orabase . Infection 1978;6:16–20.
9. De Vries-Hospers HG, Van de Waaij D. Saliva concentrations of amphotericin B following its use as an oral lozenge. Infection 1980;8:63–5.
10. Wade JC, De Jongh CA, Newman KA, Crowley J, Wiernik PH, Schimpff SC. Selective antimicrobial modulation as prophylaxis against infection during granulocytopenia: trimethoprim-sulfamethoxazole vs nalidixic acid. J Inf Dis 1983;147:624–34.
11. Kurrle E, Bhaduri S, Krieger D, Pflieger H, Heimpel H. Antimicrobial prophylaxis in acute leukemia: prospective randomized study to compare two methods of selective decontamination. Klin Wochenschrift 1983;61: 691–8.
12. Guiot HFL, Van der Meer JWM, Van Furth R. Selective antimicrobial modulation of human microbial flora: infection prevention in patients with decreased host defense mechanisms by selective elimination of potentially pathogenic bacteria. J Inf Dis 1981;143:644–54.
13. Guiot HFL, Van den Broek PJ, Van der Meer JWM, Van Furth R. Selective antimicrobial modulation of the intestinal flora of patients with acute non-lymphocytic leukemia: a double blind, placebo controlled study. J Inf Dis 1983;147:615–23.
14. De Vries-Hospers HG, Sleijfer DT, Mulder NH, Van der Waaij D, Nieweg HO, Van Saen HKF. Bacteriological aspects of selective decontamination of the digestive tract as a method of infection prevention in granulocytopenic patients. AAC 1981;19:813–20.
15. Rozenberg-Arska A, Dekker AW, Verhoef J. Colistin and trimethoprim-sulfamethoxazole for the prevention of infection in patients with acute non-lymphocytic leukemia. Decrease in the emergence of resistant bacteria. Infection 1983;11:167–9.

CMV INFECTION AND ITS PREVENTION WITH SPECIFIC IMMUNOGLOBULINS*

W.G. Ho, D.J. Winston, R.E. Champlin, R.P.Gale

Patients undergoing bone marrow transplantation for hematologic disorders are severely immunocompromised by the intensive chemotherapy and total body irradiation used in preparation for the transplant. Interstitial pneumonia occurs as a complication in approximately 40% of all bone marrow transplant recipients and is fatal in 70% of cases (1–3). Cytomegalovirus (CMV) is the most common pathogen associated with the interstitial pneumonia and can be identified in 50–70% of cases.

Attempts to treat established CMV infections with adenine arabinoside, interferon, acyclovir and combinations of these agents have proven not to be successful (4–8). Attention has therefore been focussed on the prevention of CMV infection rather than on treatment. We previously reported a controlled study of pooled cytomegalovirus immune plasma (CMVIP) in bone marrow transplant recipients (9). Although the CMVIP did not prevent CMV infection, it appeared to modify the severity of CMV infection and reduce the incidence of interstitial pneumonia. These results strongly suggested that passive immunization with CMV antibody was a useful approach to the problem. The limited availability of high titered CMV immune plasma prompted a search for alternative sources of CMV antibody. Intravenous immune globulin (immune globulin intravenous, IVIG, 5% in 10% maltose, Cutter Laboratories, Inc., Berkeley, California) with CMV antibody titers (1:30,000 by radioimmune assay) comparable to the titers in CMVIP was considered an appropriate alternative after initial pharmacokinetic, safety and toxicity studies were performed (10). This report details our preliminary experience in passive immunization of bone marrow transplant recipients with CMV immune globulin administered intravenously.

PATIENTS AND METHODS

Candidates for this study were selected from patients with leukemia or aplastic anemia admitted to the UCLA Centre for the Health Sciences for marrow transplantation. Patients were eligible if they had a pretransplant CMV complement-fixation (CF) antibody titer 1:16 and no clinical or laboratory evidence of ongoing infection. All eligible patients were randomized to receive or not to receive infusion of IVIG. The immune globulin was

* Supported by grants CA-23175, from the National Cancer Institute and by grant RR-865 from the Public Health Service. Dr. Champlin is a recipient of a New Investigator Research Award, National Institute of Arthritis, Diabetes and Kidney Disease. Dr. Gale is the Meyerhoff Visiting Scientist of the Weizman Institute of Science.

administered at a dose of 20 ml/kg pretransplant and then once every week until day + 120 posttransplant. Informed consent approved by the UCLA Human Subject Protection Committee was obtained from each patient.

Details on pretransplant conditioning therapy and posttransplant management have been reported elsewhere (11–13). Methotrexate was administered posttransplant to prevent graft-versus-host disease (GvHD) and patients who developed stage III or IV GvHD were treated with corticosteroids.

Serologic studies for cytomegalovirus antibody were performed on patients before entry into the study and then at intervals of two weeks. Cytomegalovirus antibody titers were measured by the micro titer complement-fixation test as previously described (14).

Viral cultures of throat washings, urine and buffy coat were performed on the marrow transplant recipient and then every two weeks. In addition, clinically indicated viral cultures of suspicious lesions, biopsy material and tissue obtained at autopsy were done. Samples of bone marrow, throat washings, urine and buffy coat from the marrow donor were also cultured for viruses. Cultures for CMV were performed using WI-38 monolayers for virus propagation, as well as primary monkey kidney cells. Both the mononuclear and polymorphonuclear leukocytes in buffy coats were cultured for viruses by methods previously reported (15). All cell cultures were examined twice weekly for six weeks, and viruses were identified by the range of cells infected and characteristic cytopathic effects.

Table I. Characteristics of patients.

	Control	IVIG
Patients n.	18	18
Median age (range) years	20 (4–34)	19 (6–48)
Sex, male/female n.	6/12	11/7
Underlying disease n.		
acute leukemia – remission	11	12
acute leukemia – relapse	4	2
aplastic anemia	3	4
Conditioning regimen n.		
cytoxan + total body irradiation	12	12
cytoxan + fractionated total body irradiation	3	3
fractionated total body irradiation	3	2
cytoxan	0	1
Graft-versus-host disease n.	12	9
Pretransplant CMV complement-fixation titer		
negative (< 1:8)	15	16
positive (1:8–1:16)	3	2
Marrow donor with positive CMV complement-fixation titer	2	4

RESULTS

The characteristics of the patients entered into this study are indicated in Table I. Of the 36 patients randomized, the control patients and the patients receiving IVIG were similar with respect to age, underlying disease, immunosuppressive therapy, incidence of GvHD, pretransplant CMV serologic findings, and donor CMV serologic findings. The sex ratio was reversed in the two groups of patients but the difference did not appear to be important. None of the marrow donors had positive cultures for CMV.

Infusion of IVIG produced elevations in the serum IgG level as previously described (10). As was reported previously, no CMV complement-fixation antibody could be detected above the baseline value in any of the recipients of IVG (10). The sera of these patients did not appear to be anticomplementary in the complement-fixation assay. CMV antibody titers, however, were measurable by more sensitive indirect hemagglutination radioimmune assays.

Table II. CMV infection and interstitial pneumonia.

	Control (18)	IVIG (18)
CMV infection n.	10	8
symptomatic	7 (39%)	3 (17%)
asymptomatic	3	5
Interstitial pneumonia n.	9 (50%)	4 (22%)
CMV	7	3
idiopathic	2	1
Death from interstitial pneumonia n.	8	3
Death with CMV n.	6	2

The incidences and types of CMV infections and interstitial pneumonias in the control and IVIG groups are indicated in Tabel II. Although the incidence of CMV infections was similar in both groups, symptomatic infection and interstitial pneumonia occurred less frequently in the recipients of IVIG. The difference in the incidence of interstitial pneumonia between the two groups is primarily due to a lower number of CMV-associated pneumonias among the recipients of IVIG. There was also an apparent reduction in the mortality associated with CMV in the IVIG recipients.

DISCUSSION

The preliminary results of this study suggest that passive immunization with intravenous immune globulin containing antibodies to CMV does not prevent, but modifies human CMV infection. Bone marrow transplant recipients receiving IVIG had fewer symptomatic CMV infections and a lower incidence of interstitial pneumonia. These results are similar to those reported in a previous trial of cytomegalovirus immune plasma (9).

Passive immunization of bone marrow transplant recipients has also been attempted by other investigators. Meyers et al. recently reported on the efficacy of intramuscularly administered cytomegalovirus immune globulin (16). Among patients who received no granulocyte transfusions, the recipients of immune globulin had fewer CMV infections than controls. It was concluded that CMV infection can be prevented by immunoprophylaxis in seronegative patients not given granulocyte transfusions. However, it was not clearly demonstrated that immune globulin reduced the severity of CMV infections in these patients.

In another recent study, O'Reilly et al. reported their experience in a 3-arm trial in patients receiving intravenous CMV immune globulin compared to patients receiving antibody negative globulin or nothing (17). The results suggested that passive immunization with immune globulin reduced the incidence of CMV infections, but no effect on the incidence of interstitial pneumonia was demonstrated. In this study buffy coat cultures for CMV were not performed. There was therefore a lack of sensitivity of the virus surveillance procedure, and this probably explained the apparent lack of CMV infections observed in the group receiving CMV immune globulin, especially as the globulin was administered only at approximately monthly intervals after transplantation.

From these studies it is becoming increasingly convincing that passive immunization may have a role in the prevention of CMV infection in selected bone marrow transplant recipients. At present, passive prophylaxis certainly does not provide total protection from CMV infection, at least not with antibody preparations currently available. It is clear that further studies in this direction are warranted.

REFERENCES

1. Winston DJ, Bryson YJ, Ho WG, Territo MD, Golde DW, Gale RP. Interstitial pneumonia and cytomegalovirus infection after bone marrow transplantation. In: Gale RP, Fox GE, eds. Biology of bone marrow transplantation, New York, Academic Press, 1980:83–95.
2. Winston DJ, Ho WG, Champlin RE, Gale RP. Treatment and prevention of interstitial pneumonia associated with bone marrow transplantation. In: Gale RP, Fox GE, eds. Recent advances in bone marrow transplantation. UCLA Symposia on Molecular and Cellular Biology, Vol. 7, New York: Alan R. Liss Inc. (in press).
3. Meyers JD, Flournoy N, Thomas ED. Nonbacterial pneumonia after allogeneic marrow transplantation — A review of ten years' experience. Rev Infect Dis 1982;4:1119–32.
4. Kraemer KG, Neiman PE, Reeves WC, Thomas ED. Prophylactic adenine arabinoside following marrow transplantation. Transplant Proc 1978;10:237–40.
5. Meyers JD, McGuffin RW, Neiman PE, Singer JW, Thomas ED. Toxicity and efficacy of human leukocyte interferon for treatment of cytomegalovirus pneumonia after marrow transplantation. J Infect Dis 1980;141:555–62.
6. Saral R, Burns WH, Laskin OL, Santos GW, Lietman PS. Acyclovir prophylaxis of herpes-simplex-virus infections: A randomized double blind controlled trial in bone marrow transplant recipients. N Engl J Med 1981;305:63–7.
7. Meyers JD, McGuffin RW, Bryson YJ, Cantell K, Thomas ED. Treatment of cytomegalovirus pneumonia after marrow transplant with combined vidarabine and human leukocyte interferon. J Infect Dis 1982;146:80–4.

8. Wade JC, Hintz M, McGuffin RW, Springmeyer SC, Connor JD, Meyers JD. Treatment of cytomegalovirus pneumonia with high dose acyclovir. Am J Med (Suppl) 1982;73:249–56.
9. Winston DJ, Pollard RB, Ho WG, et al. Cytomegalovirus immune plasma in bone marrow transplant recipients. Am Intern Med 1982;97:11–8.
10. Winston DJ, Ho WG, Ramussen LE, et al. Use of intravenous immune globulin in patients receiving bone marrow transplants. J Clin Immunol (Suppl) 1982;2:425–75.
11. Gale RP. Current status of bone marrow transplantation in acute leukemia. Transplant Proc 1979;9:1920–3.
12. Gale RP, Ho WG, Feig SA, Champlin RE. Prevention of graft rejection following bone marrow transplantation. Blood 1981;57:9–12.
13. Feig SA, Champlin R, Arenson E, et al. Improved survival following bone marrow transplantation in aplastic anemia. Br J Haematol 1983;54:509–17.
14. Casey HL. Adaptation of laboratory branch complement-fixation method to micro technique. Public monograph no 74 Washington DC: Government Printing Office, 1965.
15. Howell CL, Miller MJ, Martin WJ. Comparison of rates of virus isolation from leukocyte populations separated from blood by conventional and ficoll-paque/macrodex methods. J Clin Microbiol 1979;10:533–7.
16. Meyers JD, Leszczynski J, Zaia JA, et al. Prevention of cytomegalovirus infection by cytomegalovirus immune globulin after marrow transplantation. Ann Intern Med 1983;98:442–6.
17. O'Reilly RJ, Reich L, Gold J, et al. A randomized trial of intravenous hyperimmune globulin for the prevention of cytomegalovirus (CMV) infections following marrow transplantation — Preliminary results. Transplant Proc 1983;15:1405–11.

CHARACTERIZATION OF THE NEW CYTOMYGALOVIRUS IMMUNOGLOBULIN PREPARATION FOR INTRAVENOUS USE

R. Schweitzer

On the basis of the occurrence of antibodies against cytomegalovirus, the incidence of this infection in Europe and North America is about 60–70% of the total population. CMV infections are, in most cases, clinically inapparent. Alterations in the immunological defence system, caused for example by pregnancy, the presence of malignant disease, immunosuppressive or cytostatic therapy, as well as by massive transfusions of blood, are the commonest causes of an increased incidence of CMV infection, combined with a high rate of clinically overt illness (Fig. 1). This applies both to primary CMV infections as well as to the reactivation of latent virus in the body.

Primary infection	Secondary infection
(seronegative host)	(seropositive host)
mother — child	different viral serotype
transfusion	contact with infectious secretions
organ transplantation	transfusion
contact with infectious secretions	organ transplantation
	immunosuppressive therapy
	pregnancy
	Latency ⟶ reactivation

According to Weller TH 1971.

Figure 1. Pathogeneses of CMV infection.

A high rate of frequently severe and life-threatening CMV infections is observed in patients who have undergone renal, bone marrow or heart transplantation. This is due to the immunosuppression necessary to prevent organ rejection reactions. Immunosuppression favours both the reactivation of any latent CMV as well as new infections via CMV-contaminated transplants or transfusions from a CMV-antibody positive donor.

The diagnosis of an acute CMV infection is based on clinical symptoms, the virus isolation from urine or saliva, and on the serological identification of antibodies in raised titres. Great reliability in the demonstration of an acute CMV infection is attained by the identification of CMV-specific antibodies of the IgM type. IgM presence in the serum and virus excretion in urine run concomittantly during a CMV infection (Fig. 2).

As a means to bring the CMV-infection problem under control, particularly after transplants, a break-through has been achieved recently by

Isolation of virus from urine or saliva

Detection of antibodies of the IgG class by complement fixation test or hemagglutination test

Immunofluorescence test and ELISA for detection of IgG and IgM antibodies

Proof of fresh infection is given by seroconversion or 4-fold increase of the IgG anti-CMV titre

Safe proof is the detection of CMV specific IgM antibodies. Proof of IgM in serum and excretion of the virus in urine are parallel processes with CMV infection

Figure 2. Analytical methods.

passive immunization with preparations containing CMV antibodies. The results out of clinical trials reported recently suggest, that cytomegalovirus immunoglobulin effectively prevents CMV infections during the transplant period (1–4).

Biotest recently developed an cytomegalovirus immunoglobulin preparation for intravenous use (authorized since March 1983 by the Paul Ehrlich Institute for sera and vaccines) which is now available for clinical use (Fig. 3).

Method of production:

CMV immuneplasma from healthy donors; HBsAg negative; normal in serum transaminase activity
Cohn ethanol fractionation (Cohn II)
Treatment with beta-propiolactone
→ intravenous tolerance of IgG
→ inactivating effect on viruses for additonal safety
Adsorption on Aerosil®
→ removal of protein aggregates
Centrifugation and filtration
Controls

Figure 3. Cytomegalo immunoglobulin i.v. Biotest.

It is obtained from the plasma of healthy donors who show a high cytomegalovirus antibody titre. Only single plasma donations which have been tested for transaminase and absence of HB_s-antigen are used in production, according to the guidelines of the German Blood Transfusion and Immune Hematology Society.

Cytomegalovirus immunoglobulin is prepared by stabilization of the IgG antibody fraction with beta-propiolactone, using the well proven procedure for Intraglobin® (5). This process ensures excellent intravenous tolerance, as has been established in 12 years of clinical experience.

It should be noted that the beta-propiolactone step which eliminates the anticomplement activity of the intravenous immunoglobulin (IgG) preparation also provides a significant contribution to reducing the risk of transmission of any infectious agent (6).

The composition and properties of the new cytomegalovirus immunoglobulin are summarized in figures 4 and 5.

Composition:	
Protein content	10 g/100 ml
IgG content	> 95%
Anti-CMV titre	at least 50 U/ml* (1:50,000 ELISA, Biotest)
Na^+	155 mmol/l
Cl^-	155 mmol/l

* According to the standard used by the German Health Authorities (Paul Ehrlich Institute, Frankfurt/Main).

Figure 4. Cytomegalo immunoglobulin i.v. Biotest.

Properties:	
Ability for neutralization	+++
Complement activation	+++
Promotion of phagocytosis	+++
Biological half-life	18–22 days
Molecular weight	160,000 (IgG)
Anticomplementary activity	negative
I.v. tolerance	yes

Figure 5. Cytomegalo immunoglobulin i.v. biotest.

On the basis of our investigations so far and the controlled studies already carried out with other preparations, the effectiveness of cytomegalovirus immunoglobulin as a prophylactic agent is definitely established. Further controlled studies to confirm the prophylactic efficacy in bone marrow and renal transplantation are currently underway. Initial results of therapeutic trials are also promising, but further studies are envisaged.

REFERENCES

1. Condie RM, Hall BL, Howard RJ, Fry D, Simmons RL, Najarian JS. Treatment of life-threatening infections in renal transplant recipients with high-dose intravenous human IgG. Transplant Proc II 1979;1:66–8.
2. Nicholls AJ, Brown CB, Edwar N, Cuthbertson B, Yap PL, McClelland DBL. Hyperimmune immunoglobulin for cytomegalovirus infections. Lancet 1983; i:532–3.
3. O'Reilly RJ, Riech L, Gold J, et al. A randomized trial of intravenous hyperimmune globulin for the prevention of cytomegalovirus (CMV) infec-

tions following marrow transplantation: Preliminary results. IX. Intern Congress of the Transplant Society, Brighton 1982 (abstract).
4. Winston DJ, Pollard RB, Ho WG, et al. Cytomegalovirus immune plasma in bone marrow transplant recipients. Ann Intern Med 1982;97:11–8.
5. Stephan W. Undegraded human immunoglobulin for intravenous use. Vox Sang 1975;28:422–37.
6. Stephan W, Dichtelmüller H. Beta-propiolacton als sterilisierendes Agens bei der Herstellung eines intravenösen Immunoglobulin-Präparates. Arzneim Forsch/Drug Res 1983;33:1230–1.

THE ROLE OF INTERFERONS IN VIRAL INFECTIONS IN IMMUNE COMPROMISED PATIENTS*

R.T. Schooley, M.S. Hirsch, R.H. Rubin, K. Cantell

INTRODUCTION

Herpesgroup viruses remain cause of morbidity among renal allograft recipients. Over the past several years the development of antiviral drugs such as adenine arabinoside and acyclovir have resulted in major improvements in management of herpes simplex (HSV) and varicella zoster virus (VZV) infections (1). Cytomegalovirus (CMV) and Epstein-Barr virus (EBV), however, continue to contribute to the morbidity of renal transplantation (2–6). CMV infection has several effects on the host. Between 30 and 40% of all renal allograft recipients develop clinically apparent CMV syndromes and 2–3% will have fatal infections. CMV infection following transplantation may be either primary or due to reactivation of latent virus. Primary infection occurs in 60–70% of CMV seronegative renal allograft recipients who receive grafts from CMV seropositive donors. Reactivation of CMV occurs in approximately 60% of CMV seropositive recipients. Because most adult allograft recipients in the United States are CMV seropositive, primary CMV infections are less common than reactivation infections, but may be associated with more morbidity when they are observed.

Most CMV syndromes, whether primary or secondary, are noted between one and four months following transplantation. The most frequently recognized CMV syndrome following transplantation is prolonged fever. Many patients also exhibit leukopenia, thrombocytopenia or hepatitis. In some patients, CMV pneumonia will develop. Patients may recover from CMV infection or they may develop progressive disseminated infections with terminal pancytopenia, hypotension and multisystem involvement (3).

In addition to its ability to directly produce morbidity, CMV is a potent immunomodulator and may predispose the host to opportunistic infections (7). The immunomodulatory effects of CMV are diverse and include suppressive effects of CMV-infected monocytes on lymphocytes, and changes in the distribution of T-lymphocyte subsets in the peripheral blood (8,9). In association with primary and most reactivation CMV infections following transplantation, there is a relative decrease in the percentage of lymphocytes bearing the helper/inducer (OKT4) surface antigen and an increase in those bearing the cytotoxic/suppressor (OKT8) surface phenotype (10). These immunomodulatory effects may predispose the host to the opportunistic infections which not infrequently follow CMV infections in allograft recipients.

Finally, CMV has also been associated with a form of immune complex glomerulopathy (5). The mechanism by which this lesion develops is incom-

* This work was supported by grants CA12464 and AI17057 and contract N01CP-43222 from the National Institute of Health.

pletely established but the implications for the graft are significant. In our hands this lesion is associated with a 70% rate of graft loss over the ensuing six months (11). Thus CMV has at least three major deleterious effects on renal allograft recipients: direct effects of the infection, immunomodulation, and induction of glomerulopathy.

EBV reactivation is frequently observed following transplantation but is usually not clinically apparent (12). In some patients, however, EBV reactivation may be associated with leukopenia and fever for which other etiologies are not apparent. Although CMV clinically has been more frequently associated with opportunistic superinfection, EBV reactivation in renal allograft recipients is also associated with changes in peripheral blood T-lymphocyte subsets (10).

We have studied the effects of interferon in two groups of renal allograft recipients over the past eight years. These studies are the subject of this report.

METHODS

Patients

Study 1. In the initital study conducted between 1976 and 1978 adult renal allograft recipients transplanted at the Massachusetts General Hospital were eligible for inclusion in the study. After informed consent had been obtained, patients were randomized to receive placebo or interferon-alpha ($3x10^6$ U) twice weekly for 15 doses for a total of $45x10^6$ U. Patients receiving antithymocyte globulin (ATG) were randomized separately from those who did not receive ATG. All patients received azathioprine and prednisone.

Study 2. In this study patients were divided into those at risk for primary CMV infection (CMV seronegative recipients of allografts from CMV seropositive donors), or for secondary infection (CMV seropositive allograft recipients). All renal allograft recipients at risk for reactivation of CMV (anti-CMV antibody > 1:8 by indirect immunofluorescence) were eligible for inclusion in the reactivation study which was conducted at the Massachusetts General Hospital. Those at risk for primary infection were eligible for a multicentre study which is currently ongoing. Immunosuppressive regimens employed were similar to those utilized for Study 1. In Study 2, separate randomization for cadaveric and living related donors and for ATG recipients and for those who did not receive ATG was undertaken. Patients received either placebo or interferon ($3x10^6$ U) thrice weekly for six weeks, followed by twice weekly for an additional eight weeks for a total of $102x10^6$ U over 14 weeks.

Interferon. Interferon-alpha produced in short term cultures of human buffy coat leukocytes was of the partially purified (P-IF A) type (13,14). Study drug was held when the peripheral blood granulocyte count fell below $1.5x10^9$/l or the platelet count fell below $80x10^9$/l and resumed when counts improved. The study drug was discontinued if the patient underwent transplant nephrectomy within three weeks of transplantation.

Virology and serology. Samples of buffy coat leukocytes, saliva, and urine were collected at transplantation and at two weekly intervals for five months, and then at monthly intervals for seven months, processed as previously described and inoculated into human embryonic lung fibroblast monolayers (15). CMV and HSV were identified by characteristic cytopathic effect.

Saliva was also inoculated onto cord blood lymphocytes in microtiter plates. Cultures were maintained for eight weeks and observed visually for evidence of transformation. Transformed cell lines were stained for Epstein Barr nuclear antigen (EBNA) by anticomplement immunofluorescence (12,16).

Serum was allowed to clot at room temperature and then stored at -20°C until it was tested for antibodies to CMV by indirect immunofluorescent and complement fixation techniques (10). EBV antibodies were determined by indirect immunofluorescence in the laboratory of Dr. Werner Henle (17,18).

Definition of syndromes and graft failure. Cytomegalovirus syndromes were defined as illness which occurred during periods of viral excretion and rising cytomegalovirus antibody titers which had two or more of the following features: unexplained fever for at least three days, pneumonitis without other causes, leukopenia (less than $3x10^9$ white cells/l) on three or more consecutive days after discontinuation of azathioprine, elevated serum alanine aminotransferase (over 40 Karmen units) in the absence of serologic evidence of hepatitis B, and atypical lymphocytosis (over 20 percent of peripheral-blood white cells) (19). Patients were categorized as having a cytomegalovirus syndrome without knowledge of whether they were receiving interferon or placebo.

Graft failure was defined as return to permanent dialysis as a result of dysfunction induced by graft rejection or transplantation glomerulopathy. The diagnosis of cytomegalovirus-associated glomerulopathy was made in a patient whose allograft biopsy specimen obtained at the time of a 50 percent or larger decline in renal function showed the morphologic feature of the previously described glomerulopathy (6).

Opportunistic infection was defined as the occurrence of invasive infection with one or more of the following agents: L. monocytogenes, N. asteroides, candida species, aspergillus species or Mucoraceae.

Statistical analysis

Averages are expressed ± 1 SEM. Intergroup comparisons were made by the Wilcoxon-Mann-Whitney test. Proportions were compared by Fisher's exact test.

RESULTS

Study 1. In the initial study 41 adult patients were randomized to receive placebo or interferon-alpha twice weekly for six weeks. Twenty-one patients received interferon and 20 placebo. The groups were evenly matched for sex, underlying renal disease, degree of HLA match, percentage of cadaveric donors, history of blood transfusion, and number receiving ATG.

CMV excretion was delayed by interferon administration from a mean of 29 to a mean of 50 days following transplantation ($p<.03$). Among those patients who excreted CMV, CMV viremia was observed less frequently among those receiving interferon (9 of 10) than those not receiving interferon (5 of 11, $p=0.04$). CMV viremia was observed more frequently among ATG recipients, although CMV syndromes occurred more frequently among viremic patients, the trend toward fewer CMV syndromes among interferon recipients did not achieve statistical significance. EBV excretion was increased by ATG, and decreased by interferon. EBV associated leukopenia and fever was infrequent among either interferon or placebo recipients. Interferon had little demonstrable effect on HSV related excretion or morbidity.

Study 2. Because of the encouraging results encountered in the initial study, a second study was conducted in which interferon therapy was administered in higher dose, for a longer period of time. In this study patients at risk for reactivation of CMV were randomized separately from those at risk for primary infection. The primary CMV study is being conducted as a multicentre trial and is still under way.

In the reactivation study 48 patients consented to participate, but six were not analyzed because they received fewer than 10 doses of study drug. Those six patients included four who underwent early nephrectomy for acute rejection, one who received a pretransplant dose of interferon but suffered surgical complications, and one interferon recipient who refused to continue the study drug.

The remaining 42 patients were randomized into a group of 20 interferon recipients and 22 placebo recipients. The groups were well matched for age, source of kidney immunosuppressive regimens, underlying renal disease, histocompatibility match between donor and recipient, and history of blood transfusion.

CMV syndromes were reduced from 7 of 23 to 1 of 20 in placebo and interferon recipients respectively (Table I). As in our previous study CMV syndromes were more frequently observed among recipients of cadaveric kidneys who also received ATG therapy. The CMV syndromes observed included fever and leukopenia (5 patients), pneumonia (3 patients), and fever with atypical lymphocytosis (2 patients). The only CMV syndrome among interferon recipients occurred in a recipient of allograft from a living related donor who did not receive ATG. He had omitted 9 of 26 scheduled doses of interferon between the third and fourteenth week following transplantation because of thrombocytopenia.

Table I. Incidence of cytomegalovirus syndromes, according to randomization subgroup.*

Subgroup	Interferon		Placebo	Total
	no. with syndrome/no. in subgroup			
Antithymocyte globulin	0/9	p=0.02**	5/10	5/19
No antithymocyte globulin	1/11		2/12	3/23
Total	1/20	p=0.03**	7/22	8/42
Cadaver donor	0/12	p=0.01**	7/15	7/27
Living related donor	1/8		0/7	1/15
Total	1/20	p=0.03**	7/22	8/42

* Adapted with permission form The New England Journal of Medicine (20).
** By Fisher's exact test.

Only two patients developed opportunistic infections during the period of study drug administration. Both patients were placebo recipients who had become CMV infected. One patient developed disseminated aspergillosis; the other pneumocystis carinii pneumonia. CMV associated glomerulopathy was observed in three placebo and one interferon recipients during the drug administration period.

Two deaths occurred among patients in each treatment group during the drug administration period. One interferon recipient died of cardiomyopathy; the second of a perforated intestinal diverticulum. Both placebo recipients who died succumbed to infection. One patient died of cytomegalovirus pneumonia; the other patient died of cytomegalovirus and pneumocystis pneumonia. No differences in graft survival were evident six months following transplantation.

Cytomegalovirus excretion was detected slightly more frequently among placebo than interferon recipients (77 vs 60%), and was delayed by interferon among ATG recipients but not in other groups (Table II). CMV viremia was less frequently observed in this study than in the initial study being observed in only five interferon recipients and two placebo recipients (p=0.17).

Table II. Onset of urinary excretion of cytomegalovirus, according to randomization subgroup.*

Subgroup	Interferon		Placebo
	mean ± S.E.M. days after transplantation (95% confidence interval)		
Antithymocyte globulin	81±20 (42-110)	p=0.04**	50±9 (32-50)
No antithymocyte globulin	80±22 (48-123)		109±51 (30-92)
Cadaver donor	86±24 (27-110)	p=0.06**	48±8 (32-50)
Living related donor	77±16 (48-123)		126±60 (51-363)
Mean	81±15 (48-84)		75±23 (39-69)

* Adapted with permission from The New England Journal of Medicine (20).
** By Wilcoxon-Mann-Whitney test.

Interferon was extremely well tolerated by study patients in the doses used in this study. One interferon recipient withdrew from the study because of local pain at the injection site. Two interferon recipients experienced low grade fevers following interferon administration. Detectable suppressive effects on the marrow were modest. Interferon recipients missed an average of 5.2 doses of study drug because of thrombocytopenia or granulocytopenia; placebo recipients missed an average of 4.2 doses of study drug.

DISCUSSION

These studies have demonstrated virologic and clinical benefits from prophylactic interferon-alpha among renal allograft recipients at risk for CMV reactivation. Interferon delayed excretion of CMV in both studies, and prevented CMV-related morbidity in the second study which utilized higher doses of interferon over a longer period of time following transplantation. In addition to experiencing a lower incidence of clinical syndromes associated with CMV infection, interferon recipients experienced fewer opportunistic infections and a lower rate of occurrance of CMV-associated glomerulopathy.

Interferon therapy was well tolerated in both studies. Few patients experienced febrile reactions or local pain following transplantation. The drug was better tolerated from this standpoint than in other settings in which it has been utilized without concomitant prednisone and azathioprine. The marrow suppressive effects were modest and quite reversible.

Recombinant DNA technology will provide an increased supply of pure relatively inexpensive interferon preparations in the near future (21,22). The ultimate role of interferon, in the management of organ allograft recipients remains to be determined. The toxicity and optimal dosing or recombinant interferons will require study. The roles of cytomegalovirus vaccines (23), passive immunization (24), and donor selection techniques (25) are also under active study at the present time. It is likely that the proper approach to CMV related morbidity will vary from centre to centre depending on the patient populations transplanted and the immunosuppressive regimens employed. Although interferons possess activity _in vitro_ against HSV, VZV and EBV, other antiviral drugs such as acyclovir may play a greater role than interferons in management of other herpesgroup viruses (1). At the present time, interferon-alpha appears to be the best currently available approach to prevention of cytomegalovirus infections among CMV seropositive recipients of renal allografts.

REFERENCES

1. Hirsch MS, Schooley RT. Treatment of herpesvirus infections. N Engl J Med 1983;309:963.
2. Glenn J. Cytomegalovirus infections following renal transplantation. Rev Infect Dis 1981;3:1151–78.
3. Marker SC, Howard RJ, Simmons RL, et al. Cytomegalovirus infection: A quantitative prospective study of three hundred twenty consecutive renal transplants. Surgery 1981;89:660–71.
4. Harwood AR, Osoba D, Hofstader SL, et al. Kaposi's sarcoma in recipients of renal transplants. Am J Med 1979;67:759–65.
5. Richardson WP, Colvin RB, Cheeseman SH, et al. Glomerulopathy associated with cytomegalovirus viremia in renal allografts. N Engl J Med 1980; 305:57–63.
6. Hanto DW, Frizzera G, Gejl-Peczalaska J, et al. The Epstein-Barr virus in the pathogenesis of post transplant lymphoma. Transplant Proc 1981; 13:756–60.
7. Ho M. Cytomegalovirus: Biology and infection. New York, Plenum, 1982.
8. Carney WP, Hirsch MS. Mechanisms of immunosuppression in cytomegalovirus mononucleosis. II. Virus-monocyte interactions. J Infect Dis 1981;144: 47–54.

9. Carney WP, Rubin RH, Hoffman RA, Hansen WP, Healey K, Hirsch MS. Analysis of T lymphocyte subsets in cytomegalovirus mononucleosis. J Immunol 1981;126:2114–6.
10. Schooley RT, Hirsch MS, Colvin RB, et al. Association of herpesvirus infections with T-lymphocyte-subset alterations, glomerulopathy, and opportunistic infections after renal transplantation. N Engl J Med 1983;308:307–13.
11. Colvin RB, Cosimi AB, Burton RC, et al. Circulating T-cell subsets in human renal allograft recipients: The OKT4+/OKT8+ cell ratio correlates with reversibility of graft injury. Presented at the 9th International Congress of the Transplantation Society, Brighton, United Kingdom, 1982 August 23–27.
12. Cheesemen SH, Henle W, Rubin R, et al. Epstein-Barr virus infection in renal transplant recipients: Effects of antithymocyte globuline and interferon. Ann Intern Med 1980;93:39–42.
13. Cantell K, Hirvonen S, Kauppinen H-L, Myllyla G. Production of interferon in human leukocytes from normal donors with the use of Sendai virus. Methods Enzymol 1981;78:29–38.
14. Cantell K, Hirvonen S, Koistinen V. Partial purification of human leukocyte interferon on a large scale. Methods Enzymol 1981;78:499–505.
15. Cheeseman SH, Rubin RH, Stewart JA, et al. Controlled clinical trial of prophylactic human-leukocyte interferon in renal transplantation. Effects on cytomegalovirus and herpes simplex virus infections. N Engl J Med 1979;30:1345–9.
16. Reedman BM, Klein G. Cellular localization of an Epstein-Barr virus (EBV)-associated complement-fixing antigen in producer and non-producer lymphoblastoid cell lines. Int J Cancer 1973;11:499–520.
17. Henle G, Henle W. Immunofluorescence in cells derived from Burkitt's lymphoma. J Bacteriol 1966;91:1248–56.
18. Henle G, Henle W, Klein G. Demonstration of two distinct components in the early antigen complex of Epstein-Barr virus-infected cells. Int J Cancer 1971;8:272–82.
19. Rubin RH, Cosimi AB, Tolkoff-Rubin NE, Russell PS, Hirsch MS. Infectious disease syndromes attributable to cytomegalovirus and their significance among renal transplant recipients. Transplantation 1977; 24:458–64.
20. Hirsch MS, Schooley RT, Cosimi AB, et al. Effects of interferon-alpha on cytomegalovirus reactivation syndromes in renal-transplant recipients. N Engl J Med 1983;308:1489–93.
21. Horning SJ, Levine JF, Miller RA, Rosenberg SA, Merigan TC. Clinical and immunologic effects of recombinant leukocyte A interferon in eight patients with advanced cancer. JAMA 1982;247:1718–22.
22. Scott GM, Phillpotts RJ, Wallace J, Gauci CL, Greiner J, Tyrrell DAJ. Prevention of rhinovirus colds by human interferon alpha-2 from _Escherichia coli_. Lancet 1982;ii:186–8.
23. Starr SE, Glazer JP, Friedman HM, Farquhar JD, Plotkin SA. Specific cellular and humoral immunity after immunization with live Towne strain cytomegalovirus vaccine. J Infect Dis 1981;143:585–9.
24. Zaia JA, Levin MJ, Leszczynski J, Wright GG, Grady GF. Cytomegalovirus immune globulin: production from selected normal donor blood. Transplantation 1979;27:66–7.
25. Andrus CH, Betts RF, May AG, Freeman RB. Cytomegalovirus infection blocks the beneficial effect of pretransplant blood transfusion on renal allograft survival. Transplantation 1979;28:451–6.

FUNDAMENTALS OF PLATELET AND GRANULOCYTE SUPPORT IN MYELOSUPPRESSED LEUKEMIA AND BONE MARROW TRANSPLANT PATIENTS*

J.P. Hester, R. Ayyar, M. Keating, K. Dicke

INTRODUCTION

The basic objective of platelet replacement is to provide hemostasis for patients with inadequate bone marrow function who are at risk for major and/or fatal hemorrhage from thrombocytopenia. The degree of physiologic deficit generally accepted to correlate with an increased risk of hemorrhage is a peripheral blood platelet concentration $< 20 \times 10^9/l$. In general, a normal template bleeding time is believed to reflect in vivo hemostasis. The fundamental task would appear to be to: 1) establish the relationship between peripheral blood platelet concentration and a normal bleeding time; and 2) define the total dose of cells required to achieve this concentration. The intravascular survival of the transfused platelets would then determine the frequency of replacement and the duration of myeolosuppression would define the total number of transfusions required. However, biologic systems do not lend themselves to such simple solutions and complications in interpretation of transfusion results occur from numerous patient and component variables. Transfusion response is altered by numerous clinical variables which may occur as single events or combinations of events. Issues related to the component include the selection of pooled units of platelet concentrates versus single donor, and fresh versus stored platelets. Issues relating to granulocyte concentrates include all those enumerated for platelet replacement, but introduce unresolved questions of identifying patients whose infections will not be controlled by antibiotics alone and defining response criteria.

It is this perplexing mass of interrelated questions which must be resolved to bring rationality to component support. This report will focus on two areas: 1) quantitating the basic dose-response relationships in platelet replacement which correlate with hemostasis and defining a model for intravascular survival of transfused platelets and 2) correlating infectious and hemorrhagic events with final response to induction chemotherapy in acute leukemia patients, which should reflect adequacy of hemostatic support and antibiotic management of infections. It is beyond the scope of this paper to quantitatively define the contribution of individual clinical variables to platelet transfusion response. That is, alloimmunization, infection, hemorrhage, consumption coagulopathies, and splenic sequestration.

* Supported in part by grant CA28153 from the Public Health Service, Department of Health Education, and Welfare, National Cancer Institute, National Institutes of Health, Bethesda, Maryland.

MATERIALS AND METHODS

One-hundred ninety-two patients with previously untreated acute leukemia were registered on primary chemotherapy induction regimens. Multiagent antibiotic regimens were initiated with neutropenic patients ($< 0.5 \times 10^9/l$) had sustained temperature elevations $\geq 38°C$, and were changed as indicated by identification of infecting organisms and antibiotic sensitivity. Platelet concentrates were transfused when peripheral blood platelet counts were in the range of $20 \times 10^9/l$. Platelet concentrates were collected from related or unrelated donors using the IBM 2997 dual stage channel and were transfused as fresh or 24 hour stored concentrates. Pooled units of platelets, fresh to 72 hour stored were obtained from usual Blood Bank sources and were transfused when single donor concentrates were unavailable. The total number of platelets transfused ($\times 10^{11}$) was determined from volume and concentration measurements of all single donor concentrates. Platelet yields were not available for all pooled unit concentrates, but mean yields were established from measurements of 50 transfusions of pooled units. Patient blood volume estimates were established from height and weight models (1), 60–90 minute post-transfusion then daily platelet counts were obtained and the post-transfusion increment and percent recovery were calculated as follows:

$$\text{Expected increment } (I_E) = \frac{\text{Total platelets transfused } \times 10^{11}}{\text{Recipient blood volume (L)}}$$

$$\text{Observed increment } (I_O) = \text{Post-pretransfusion platelet concentration}$$

$$\text{Percentage recovery} = I_O / I_E$$

Splenic sequestration is variable (2,3) so adjustments in increment and recovery using standard "correction factors" were not used in order to minimize inaccuracies in interpretation. Template bleeding time determinations were made pre- and post-transfusion for 33 patients.

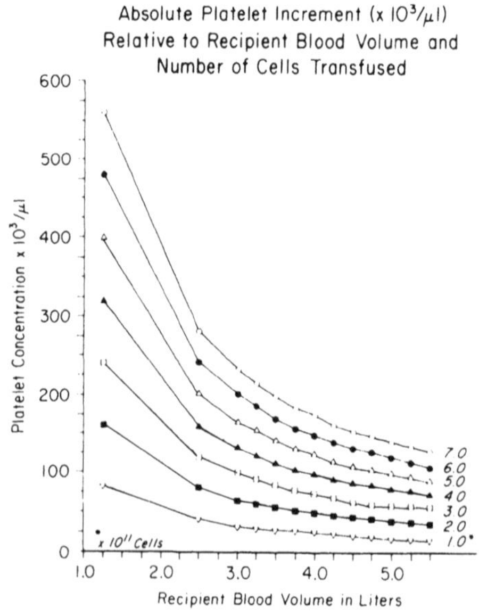

Figure 1.

RESULTS

Platelet recovery post-transfusion

The transfusion physiology of all components indicates that the post-transfusion concentration is directly correlated with cell dose and inversely related to blood volume. Variability in the number of platelets collected and recipient blood volume estimates exists in every transfusion event. The simplest of all calculations would be to calculate the expected increment per liter if all the transfused platelets circulated in the recipient's peripheral blood. The relationship between cell dose, recipient blood volume and expected platelet increment is shown in Figure 1, for a range of cell doses and blood volume estimates. An important reference calculation is that $1.0x10^{11}/l$ blood volume would be expected to give a platelet concentration of $100x10^{9}/l$.

Table I. Recipient response to transfusion with dual stage platelet concentrates.

Mean total platelets transfused $x10^{11}$ cells	= 3.8	
Mean recipient blood volume + collect volume	= 4.5 l	
Expected increment (I_E)	$= \frac{3.8x10^{11}}{4.5x10^{3}\ ml}$	$= 83x10^{9}/l$
Observed increment (I_O)	$= 34x10^{9}/l$	
Percentage recovery	$= \frac{I_O}{I_E}$	= 41%

Table I summarizes the response of 70 patients to 312 transfusions of fresh single donor concentrates. It demonstrates that the observed increment varies widely, is being modified by many factors and represents an average recovery of 41% of the cells transfused.

Bleeding time correction

In vivo platelet function, as measured by template bleeding time, was measured in thirty-three patients pre- and post-transfusion and correlated with absolute platelet concentrations (4). The mean pre-transfusion platelet count was 22 ± $11x10^{9}/l$, and the mean template bleeding time was 16.1 ± 7.7 minutes. The mean post-transfusion platelet count was 49 ± $25x10^{9}/l$ with a mean bleeding time of 7.5 ± 5.5 minutes, levels which differed significantly from pre-transfusion values ($p<.01$). In previous studies of normal donors in our laboratory (5), a normal bleeding time of 7.5 ± 2.5 minutes was established. To establish that a correlation between bleeding time and platelet count existed, the data was then analyzed relative to bleeding time measurements which were less or greater than one standard

Table II. Recipient template bleeding time and platelet count pre- and post-transfusion.

	1 SD <	Mean	> 1 SD
Pre-transfusion BT (min)	7.4	16.1	24.8
Platelet $x10^9/l$ patients	29 ± 10 (6)	21 ± 11 (21)	11 ± 6 (6)
Post-transfusion BT (min)	2.0	7.5	12
Platelet $x10^9/l$ patients	- -	55 ± 23 (28)	24 ± 10 (5)

deviation from the mean, pre- and post-transfusion. As shown in Table II, 27/33 (82%) patients had a prolonged bleeding time and a platelet count averaging $21x10^9/l$ prior to transfusion. Twenty-eight patients had a corrected bleeding time post-transfusion which correlated with the increment achieved post-transfusion. Five patients who failed to show bleeding time corrections also failed to achieve a significant post-transfusion increment.

Intravascular survival of platelets

The question of expected survival and the rate of disappearance of transfused platelets from the intravascular space is also complex. Though many studies indicate an 8–10 day survival of isotope-labeled autologous platelets, survival of transfused platelets, at least in clinically important quantities, is less and a standard reference curve against which transfused concentrates can be compared does not exist.

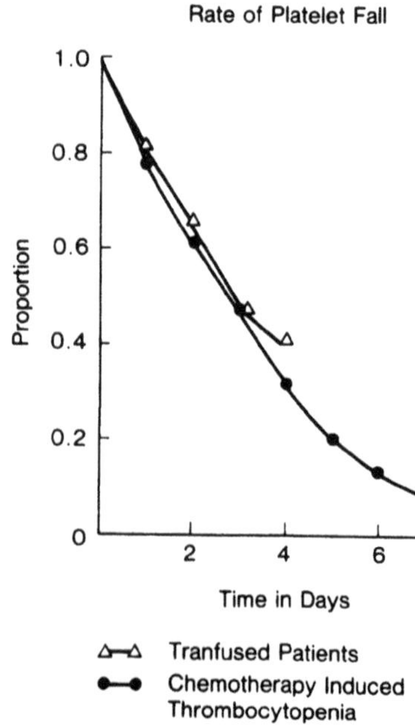

Figure 2.

A rather simple model for characterizing the rate of platelet loss is that of acute leukemia patients in remission whose peripheral blood platelet counts are often in excess of 600×10^9/l and whose bone marrow production is transiently interrupted by courses of chemotherapy. The rate of fall in platelet counts fell from a mean of 460×10^9/l to 24×10^9/l in eight days. Using the one hour post-transfusion platelet count as the baseline, the rate of platelet fall was measured in sixty transfusions of fresh single donor concentrates to patients without infection or hemorrhage. The rate of fall of the transfused concentrates was comparable to that observed in patients with chemotherapy-induced marrow suppression, as shown in Figure 2. The mean pre-transfusion platelet count was 20×10^9/l, rose to 70×10^9/l one hour post-transfusion and at 96 hours had fallen to 29×10^9/l.

The absolute counts and the rate of fall, then, described quatitatively the duration of hemostasis and predict the interval between transfusions. Further analyses are underway to determine whether clinical or component variables are associated with reduced recovery and/or accelerated rates of platelet loss and whether quantitative comparisons can be made using this model.

Granulocyte recovery post-transfusion

The absolute post-transfusion granulocyte increment and recovery are significantly lower than that achieved in platelet transfusion because of the lower dose transfused and leukocyte kinetics. However, the observed granulocyte increment is also directly related to the dose transfused, as shown in Figure 3, and inversely related to recipient blood volume. Granulocyte recovery is also influenced by the kinetic properties of granulocytes. Leukocyte

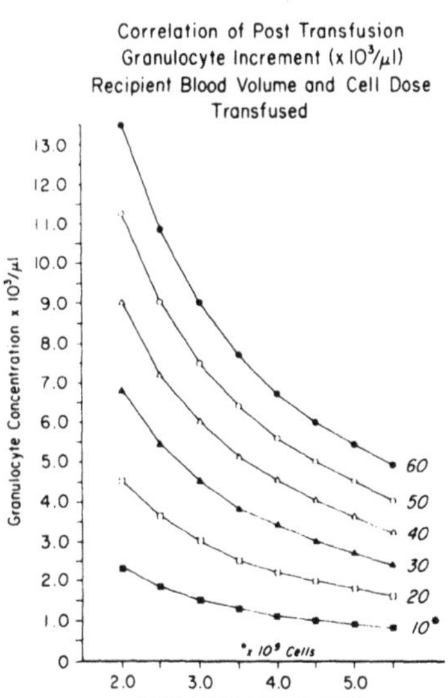

Figure 3.

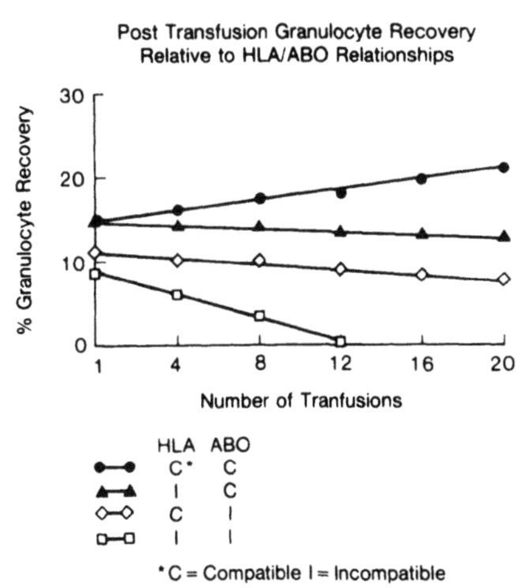

Figure 4.

kinetics indicate that there are essentially two "pools" of granulocytes, a circulating pool and a marginated pool and 56% in the marginating pool. Present methods do not allow precise measurement of the rate of egress of granulocytes into the tissues and areas of infection, so correction for these two factors are not usually made. There are also statistically significant relationships between granulocyte recovery and histocompatibility ($p<.05$) and ABO compatibility ($p<.005$) of donor recipient pairs, and the number of transfusions received, as shown in Figure 4 from an analysis of 980 granulocyte transfusions. It can also be observed that granulocyte recovery is significantly less than platelet recovery, even when ABO-HLA compatibility exists between donor recipient pairs. For the purpose of this study, HLA compatibility was defined as sharing by donors and recipients of all four A and B locus antigens.

Table III. Variables relating to response to primary induction – acute leukemia patients.

	Remission evaluation	
	Complete remission	Fail
Variable	Number of patients (%)	Number of patients (%)
All patients	118 (61%)	74 (39%)
Age – Years		
< 50	77 (67%)	38 (33%)
> 50	41 (53%)	36 (47%)
Hemorrhage		
yes	16 (35%)	30 (65%)
no	101 (73%)	36 (27%)
Infection		
FUO	55 (80%)	13 (20%)
sepsis	26 (67%)	13 (23%)
pneumonia	22 (50%)	22 (50%)
p + s	7 (26%)	20 (74%)

Table IV. Clinical characteristics of acute leukemia patients failing in the first 60 days.

	Causes of death		
	Hemorrhage	Hemorrhage + Infection	Infection
Patients	6 (14%)	22 (52%)	14 (33%)
Median survival time – days	21	12	18
Range	3–59	3–60	1–56

Impact of infection and hemorrhage on remission

Historically, infection and hemorrhage (6) have been significantly associated with failure to achieve complete remission in primary induction acute leukemia patients. Management of infection in myelosuppressed patients has been primarily directed toward development of more effective antibiotic regimens and the use of reverse or completely sterile isolation. The use of granulocyte replacement has diminished considerably as issues of patient selection, effective cell dose, response criteria and donor toxicity could not be resolved. To evaluate the effectiveness of current antibiotic and platelet replacement strategies, the records of 192 acute leukemia patients were analyzed to establish the incidence of major hemorrhage and/or infection and whether these clinical events influenced the remission response.

Complete remission was achieved in 118 (61%) patients and was not influenced by leukemic diagnosis (myeloblastic versus non-myeloblastic), patient sex, or protective isolation. Complete remission rates were negatively influenced by patient age, major hemorrhage, the presence of pneumonia and septicemia or pneumonia alone, but not isolated sepsis, fever of unknown origin, as shown in Table III. Resistant leukemia, as a cause of failure was observed in 10% of patients.

Major hemorrhage, defined as cerebrovascular, pulmonary or gastrointestinal, was observed in forty-six patients, thirty of whom (65%) failed to enter remission. Of these thirty patients, twenty-three had received only pooled platelet unit replacement, and their median survival time of 24 days was significantly less ($p<.01$) than the seven patients who received single donor platelet concentrates, whose median survival was 58 days.

Infection and hemorrhage, as causes of death, may be independent or associated events. Forty-two patients died in the first 60 days of induction chemotherapy. Table IV summarizes the causes of death and survival time, and indicates that 14% of patients died of hemorrhage alone, 52% of hemorrhage and infection, and 33% of infection alone. These data suggest that remission rates continue to be influenced by these two events and that replacement strategies still need to be modified.

DISCUSSION

Some nineteen years after the clinical effectiveness of platelet and/or granulocyte replacement has been established, many variables which influence the transfusion event have not been quantitatively characterized, and therapy strategies for these two components of blood has lagged behind red cell replacement. This relates in part to the more complex technology required to collect these concentrates, their limited storage life, the lack of a clinically useful typing system outside ABO, Rh, and histocompatibility typing, and the inability to clearly define response criteria, especially for granulocyte concentrates. Granulocyte replacement is still considered to represent a secondary supplemental therapy to be used only when primary antibiotic management has failed.

It is perhaps important to briefly summarize the historical aspects of platelet and granulocyte replacement which have relevance to development of transfusion strategies today. The physiological deficit in peripheral blood granulocyte count ($\leq 1.0 \times 10^9$/l) and platelet concentrations ($\leq 20 \times 10^9$/l) which was associated with increased risks of infection and hemorrhage have been established. These were defined by Freireich in 1966 (7) and remain the reference value for initiation of antibiotics for infection and platelet transfusions. The literature was not clear, however, as to the number of platelets which should be transfused to achieve hemostasis. Djerassi and Farber had reported in 1963 (8) that although there was inherent variability in the incidence and course of hemorrhage in thrombocytopenic patients, hemostasis was most consistently apparent in patients whose post-transfusion platelet count was increased by $40 \times 10^9/l$. This observation was not apparently pursued, but the correlation of in-vivo bleeding time correction and post-transfusion increments averaging $40 \times 10^9/l$ in the study reported here would appear to add confirmation to this historical observation. One of the factors which may have obscured dose-response relationships was reporting recipient response in terms of increment/unit transfused/m^2 without measuring the numerical quantity being transfused. An additional factor which may have complicated transfusion response is reducing the expected increment by one third to account for splenic sequestration. As reported by Simon and Murphy in 1983 (2), the range in recovery of autologous labeled platelets was 40 to 80%, with the average appearing to be about 57%. Buchholz (3) reported a mean recovery of 70% in autologous labeled platelets, with a range from 56 to 101%, suggesting errors in evaluation of platelet response may occur as a result of using a constant "correction factor".

Immunological considerations in transfusion are also broad and not clearly defined. The need for ABO compatibility of donor-recipient pairs when red cell contamination was present in platelet concentrates was suggested by Aster in 1965 (9), based on decreased recovery of labeled platelets in ABO incompatible transfusion, but this observation, too, was not pursued. The development of continuous flow techniques (IBM 2997 and CS3000) which limit red cell cross-cellular contamination may remove this factor from consideration for most transfusions. It is not known whether red cell isoagglutinins present in donor plasma may have any role in platelet transfusion.

Yankee (10) recognized the relevance of the HLA typing system in identifying related compatible donor-recipient pairs and the same observations were subsequently made for unrelated pairs. Because of the difficulty in finding HLA compatible unrelated donors, Duquesnoy (11) investigated and reported the feasibility of identifying donors with lesser degrees of compatibility. Aster (12) has concluded that satisfactory response is achieved with donor-recipient pairs mismatched by HLA antigens that are serologically cross-reactive with eachother, that mismatching at the C locus is usually of no consequence, but statistical correlations which could confirm this were not reported. More recently, Schiffer (13) reported that when 2740 HLA typed donors were screened as potential donors for alloimmunized patients, only 1.3 donors perfectly matched could be identified for each patient. He also indicated that 30–50% of HLA matched transfusions are ineffective, including a variable number of "A" matches. Schiffer and Slichter (14) also suggest that refractoriness to antibodies directed solely against platelet-specific antigens might be increased from the use of HLA matched platelets. They reported that animals receiving platelets from DLA matched littermates (the dog leukocyte antigen equivalent to HLA) became immunized.

The influence of immunological factors in platelet transfusion is also linked to issues of selection of single donor versus random pooled platelets. The inability to predict who will and who will not become immunized, or the number of transfusions, or length of time to immunization, what antigen typing is the most relevant, leaves this issue unresolved at present.

The relevance of HLA donor-recipient compatibility to granulocyte transfusion was first established in 1972 by Graw (15), the number of granulocyte transfusions which correlated with infection control by McCredie et al. (16), and the relevance of transfusion of at least 20×10^9 cells to response was reported by Vogler in 1978 (17). Two of these factors (dose and donor-patient compatibility) may have played a significant role in the negative study reported in 1981 from a controlled trial of prophylactic granulocyte transfusions during chemotherapy induction for acute leukemia (18). Unrelated as well as related donors were selected in this multi-institutional trial, but HLA matching or antibody testing prior to transfusion were not reported. Seventy-two percent of transfused patients had transfusion reactions, and 35% of transfused patients who developed pulmonary reactions died during the study compared to 5% of patients without pulmonary infiltration. The dose of granulocytes transfused averaged $3.4 \times 10^9/m^2$, suggesting that less than 10×10^9 granulocytes were received by many patients.

Other issues relevant to the use of granulocytes relate to questions of transmission of infections such as CMV. Ho et al. (19) reported that recipients of granulocyte transfusions had a higher incidence of CMV infections than untransfused patients. Donor response to macromolecular sedimenting agents and possible toxicity has also had impact on decreasing granulocyte utilization. New guidelines to limit donation using current high molecular weight hydroxyethyl starch will be forthcoming (20). However, Phase I studies of a low molecular weight hydroxyethyl starch specifically formulated for granulocyte donors has been completed (Hester, unpublished data) and Phase II multi-institutional trials are underway. This should allow renewed considerations for the use of granulocyte concentrations which will: 1) permit more specific identification of patients and types of infection which might benefit from granulocyte replacement with exclusion of patients expected to respond to antibiotic management alone, 2) assure pharmacological safety for donors following multiple donations, and 3) permit re-examination of issues relating to identification of compatible donors and cell dose-response curves.

REFERENCES

1. Mollison PL. Blood transfusion in clinical medicine. London: Blackwell Scientific, 1983:99–128.
2. Simon TL, Nelson EJ, Carmen R, Murphy S. Extension of platelet concentrate storage. Transfusion 1983;23:207–12.
3. Buchholz DH, Porten JH, Menitove JE, et al. Description and use of the CS-3000 blood cell separator for single donor platelet collection. Transfusion 1983;23:190–6.
4. Hester JP, McCredie KB, Freireich EJ. Response to chronic leukapheresis procedures and survival of chronic myelogenous leukemia patients. Transfusion 1982;22:305–7.
5. Roper PR. The relationship between age, volume, and function in the human platelet population. A dissertation for the degree of Doctor of Philosophy, The University of Texas Health Science Center at Houston, 1978.
6. Estey E, Keating MJ, Body GP, McCredie KB, Freireich EJ. Causes of failure of remission induction in actue myelogenous leukemia (AML). Proc Amer Soc Clin Oncol 1980;21:436.

7. Gaydos LA, Freireich EJ, Mantel N. The quantitative relationship between platelet count and hemorrhage in patients with acute leukemia. N Engl J Med 1962;266:905–9.
8. Djerassi I, Farber S. Control and prevention of hemorrhage: Platelet transfusion. Cancer Res 1964;25:1499–504.
9. Aster R. Effect of anticoagulant and ABO compatibility on recovery of transfused human platelets. Blood 1965;26:732–44.
10. Yankee RA. Importance of histocompatibility in platelet therapy. Vox Sang 1971;20:419–26.
11. Duquesnoy RJ, Filip DJ, Aster RH. Influence of HLA-A2 on the effectiveness of platelet transfusions in alloimmunized thrombocytopenic patients. Blood 1977;50:407–12.
12. Aster RH. Matching of blood platelets for transfusion. Am J Hemat 1978; 5:373–8.
13. Schiffer CA, Keller C, Dutcher JP, Aisner J, Hogge D, Wiernik PH. Potential HLA-matched platelet donor availability for alloimmunized patients. Transfusion 1983;23:286–9.
14. Schiffer CA, Slichter SJ. Platelet transfusions from single donors. N Engl J Med 1982;307:245–6.
15. Graw RG, Herzig G, Henderson PS. Normal granulocyte transfusion therapy. Treatment of septicemia due to gram negative sepsis. N Engl J Med 1972; 287:367.
16. McCredie KB, Freireich EJ, Hester JP, Vallejos C. Leukocyte transfusion therapy for patients with host-defense failure. Transplant Proc 1973;5: 1285–9.
17. Vogler WR, Winton EF, Larson DH. Methods of collection and results of transfusion of granulocytes. Exp Hematol 1978;6:93.
18. Strauss RG, Connett JE, Gale RP, et al. A controlled trial of prophylactic granulocyte transfusions during initial induction chemotherapy for acute myelogenous leukemia. N Engl J Med 1981;305:597–603.
19. Winston DS, Ho WG, Young LS. Prophylactic granulocyte transfusions during human bone marrow transplantation. Am J Med 1980;68:893–7.
20. Mishler JM, Hester JP, Huestis D, Rock G, Strauss RG. Dosage and scheduling regimens for erythrocyte sedimenting macromolecules. J Clin Apheresis. In press, 1983.

THE USE OF MONOCLONAL ANTIBODIES IN CLINICAL TRANSPLANTATION

G. Opelz

INTRODUCTION

With the introduction of monoclonal antibodies by Köhler and Milstein (1), both basic and clinical immunology have moved into a new era of fascinating new opportunities. Thus far, the basic scientists have been the primary beneficiaries. Antibodies of absolute purity and specificity allow the in vitro characterization of, and interaction with, specific molecules of the immunologically reactive cell. The antibodies are of such delicate specificity that different monoclonal antibodies can react with different epitopes of the same molecule, without steric hindrance. The in vivo application in experimental animals provided new insights into various immuno-regulatory mechanisms. Clinical medicine is beginning to utilize monoclonal antibodies as a diagnositc tool and, in first carefully controlled studies, the feasibility of their therapeutic use is being explored.

Transplantation immunologists are concerned particularly with cellular immune reactivity against transplanted tissue (or against the host in the case of bone marrow transplants). The identification, characterization, and specific in vivo manipulation of certain cell populations with monoclonal antibodies, therefore, is especially important in this field.

The use of monoclonal antibodies in clinical organ transplantation is still in its infancy. However, progress has been rapid and is accelerating. This attempt to summarize the current state of the art will likely be outdated by the time it is printed.

WHAT ARE MONOCLONAL ANTIBODIES?

By definition, monoclonal antibodies are produced by a clone derived from a single cell. This provides a key advantage over "conventional" antibodies (for example, antibodies produced in a rabbit or a mouse in response to injected human lymphocytes, which are the product of many different cells): their reactivity is specific in the purest immunological sense. Antibodies directed against a given antigen, e.g. an antigen that is present on the surface of T lymphocytes, do not contain "contaminating" antibodies against other antigenic substances in human blood.

Most monoclonal antibodies in use today are of mouse origin. Why is it then that "conventional" mouse antibodies against human lymphocytes are impure and crossreact with other antigens, whereas mouse-monoclonal antibodies are not? The state of purity is obtained through special manipulation of antibody producing mouse cells. Let us return to the example of a mouse-anti-human T cell antibody. If we inject a mouse with human lymphocytes, it will produce a variety of antibodies against many different antigens; among them will be antibodies against the T cell antigen that we are interested in. By means of absorption and elution, etc., we can obtain antibodies that are relatively specific. However, they usually crossreact with several antigens when sensitive assays are employed. This problem can be circumvented by selecting one single antibody producing cell, culturing it in vitro, and collecting the antibodies that it produces. Each cell produces antibodies of only one specificity which eliminates the need for absorption. Because each individual cell produces a very small quantity of antibodies, it is necessary to enhance antibody production by cloning the cell, thus increasing antibody production by multiplying the number of producing cells. Technical details how this is achieved can be found in the literature (2). Briefly, mice are immunized with antigen, mouse spleen cells are obtained and fused in vitro with mouse myeloma cells. The fused cells (hybrids) are cultured and the culture supernatants are screened for antibody reactivity against the immunizing antigen. When antibodies are found, the cell suspensions are diluted to obtain single-cell cultures. A cell clone originating from a single antibody producing cell will produce antibodies of a single specificity. Finally, once a producing clone is obtained, the antibody producing cells can be injected intraperitoneally into a mouse, which yields ascites rich in monoclonal antibodies.

MONOCLONAL ANTIBODIES RELEVANT TO CLINICAL TRANSPLANTATION

Of particular interest are monoclonal antibodies which react with cells of the immune system. The most frequently used commercially available antibodies are listed in Table I. It is interesting to note that different nomenclatures are used in the literature and that the often cited ratio of helper lymphocytes : suppressor lymphocytes may be called "4/8 ratio" or "3/2 ratio", depending on the investigator's preference. Essentially, the different commercial products' reactivity is comparable (3). The listing in Table I is

Table I. Commonly used monoclonal antibodies.

Cell type	Ortho	Becton-Dickinson	Coulter
Pan-T lymphocytes	OKT3 (OKT1)	Leu4 (Leu1)	T101
T-helper lymphocytes	OKT4	Leu3	T4
T-suppressor/cytotoxic lymphocytes	OKT8	Leu2	T8
Thymocytes	OKT6	Leu6	
B lymphocytes and monocytes activated T cells	OKTa1	Leu12	
Adherent mononuclear	OKM1		
Precursors	OKT10		
E-rosette receptor	OKT11	Leu5	T11
NK (Natural killer)		Leu11	

Table II. Functional characteristics (simplified).

	OKT4+ Leu3+	OKT8+ Leu2+
MLC response	+	-
Antigen response proliferative	+	-
Helper/inducer	+	-
Release of mitogenic and helper factors	+	-
Suppression of B cell response	-	+
Cytotoxic cells	-	+

Complex regulatory circuits.

by no means complete; many antibodies of identical or similar specificity, and of specificities characterizing additional cell subtypes, have been produced by various investigators. Table I lists the reagents that are most widely used and most frequently cited in the literature.

Most clinical investigations have been done with antibodies directed against pan-T, T-helper, and T-suppressor cells. Phenotypic identification of functionally different T cell subsets has become a widely used procedure. The essential functional differences between helper and suppressor/cytotoxic cells are listed in Table II. Apparently, complex regulatory circuits exist within the immune system, maintaining a delicate balance. New functional characteristics of known cell types are still being discovered. For example, the OKT4-positive helper cells may block suppressor circuits under certain experimental conditions. A complex and complicated picture of cellular immunity is emerging as monoclonal antibodies allow the exploration of intricate cell-to-cell interactions.

USE OF MONOCLONAL ANTIBODIES IN CLINICAL BONE MARROW TRANSPLANTATION

Utilization of monoclonal antibodies has included monitoring of cellular reconstitution following marrow transplantation, in vivo application for the treatment of GvHD (graft-versus-host disease), and in vitro treatment of marrow prior to transplantation in order to eliminate T lymphocytes or leukemic cells.

A successful marrow transplant must reconstitute the recipient's immune system. With monoclonal antibodies it is possible to follow the gradual return of "normal" cell populations in the recipient, although the cells may not yet be fully functional. Interestingly, there is an imbalance in the occurrence of different subpopulations, with an initial increase of cells carrying the suppressor phenotype (4–7). Later in the course of the transplant the imbalance of helper/ suppressor cells is reduced. Whether regulatory mechanisms are operative that are important for the fate of the graft, is being studied. Some investigators found evidence that alterations in cell phenotypes correlated with the occurrence of GvHD (4), whereas others did not (5,6).

The in vivo treatment of GvHD with anti-T cell antibodies has not been successful thus far. Although the clinical symptoms of GvHD were improved, the improvement was only temporary. In vivo administration of the anti-T cell antibody "64.1" resulted in the development of polyclonal B cell lymphomas of donor cell origin in two patients treated in Seattle (8). Possibly, the massive suppression of T cells may have eliminated the regulatory forces necessary to prevent uncontrolled proliferation of B cells.

Emphasis has therefore shifted towards in vitro treatment of marrow with anti-T cell antibodies prior to transplantation. The rationale for this is based on experimental animal data, in which prevention of GvHD was obtained regularly following the in vitro depletion of T cells (9–11). Initial clinical results with anti-T preincubated marrow showed a dramatic reduction in the occurrence of GvHD. However, a significant fraction of patients still developed GvHD (12–14). It was speculated that the mechanism required for the depletion of antibody-coated cells in vivo, namely opsonization and subsequent elimination via the reticulo-endothelial system, may be deficient in marrow transplant patients who are pretreated with irradiation or massive doses of immunosuppressive drugs. Recently, marrow preincubation with anti-T cell antibodies plus rabit complement was introduced, thereby eliminating T cells by complement dependent cytotoxic lysis in vitro, rather than via in vivo opsonization. Preliminary results in some 40 patients transplanted in this manner in Seattle, Minneapolis, and Madison suggest that a further reduction in the incidence of GvHD can be achieved.

As the depletion of T cells from marrow prior to transplantation reduces the risk of GvHD, perfect histocompatibility may become a less stringent requirement for bone marrow transplantation. Until now, the vast majority of successful marrow grafts have been done from HLA-identical sibling donors. Now that the obstacle of GvHD seems to become controllable, HLA non-identical transplants may become a viable alternative for patients who do not have an HLA-identical sibling donor (15).

Finally, promising results have been obtained with the in vitro pretreatment of leukemic marrow prior to transplantation with anti-leukemic monoclonal antibodies (16). Perhaps this new form of transplantation, whereby the patient's own leukemic bone marrow is treated in vitro, thereby depleting malignant cells, and an autologous transplant is performed following intensive anticancer medication (otherwise lethal because of marrow toxicity), will prove to be the most important application of monoclonal antibodies in clinical bone marrow transplantation.

USE OF MONOCLONAL ANTIBODIES IN CLINICAL KIDNEY TRANSPLANTATION

Monitoring of lymphocyte subpopulations following renal transplantation for the early diagnosis and characterization of immune reactions has evolved into a routine procedure at many transplant centres. Cosimi and coworkers were first to report that clinical rejection usually is preceded by an increase in the T-helper/T-suppressor cell ratio (17). These findings were confirmed by many investigators (18–21), although others questioned the practical usefulness of lymphocyte subset monitoring (22,23). A consensus is emerging that the simple enumeration of lymphocyte subpopulations at any given time is not very useful. There is too much variation in the results to allow a valid interpretation from one reading. Changes in the immunosuppressive regimen that the patient receives and infections cause fluctuations, and sometimes there are fluctuations without apparent reason (24,25). In our own experience, subset monitoring is meaningful only if performed repeatedly, allowing a comparison of serial readings.

The recognition that a simple increase in the T-helper/T-suppressor ratio is not necessarily synonymous with rejection has resulted in a more differentiated evaluation of subset monitoring results. For example, Colvin et al. pointed out that subset measurements appear to correlate with reversibility of rejection (26). Others stressed the importance of characterizing rejections by identifying the infiltrating cell populations with monoclonal antibodies (27). The important finding that helper/suppressor ratios reverse during viral infection (28,29) is used in the clinic to appropriately adapt immunosuppression. A patient with an elevated creatinine level is not given higher doses of immunosuppression if an inverted helper/suppressor ratio suggests that a viral infection may be the cause. Of course, to increase immunosuppression in an infected patient would be quite wrong and endanger the patient's life. On the other hand, if a rise in creatinine coincides with an increase in the helper/suppressor ratio, immunologic rejection is likely taking place and immunosuppression must be intensified.

Our data show a striking correlation of graft survival with lymphocyte subset changes in patients who are on a protocol of prophylactic rabbit-anti-human anti-thymocyte globulin (ATG). Among 34 patients who received a 14-day course of ATG, those whose T helper lymphocytes increased showed a high rate of rejection crises immediately following termination of ATG treatment (Table III). The data indicate that certain patients' lymphocyte escape from the immunosuppressive effect of ATG. The identification of patients who do not respond adequately to ATG as shown by subset monitoring will reduce the danger of losing their grafts.

Table III. OKT4 + lymphocytes during 14-day course of ATG.

	Rejection Crisis	No Rejection Crisis
OKT4 + increase	14	2
OKT4 + decrease	3	15 $< p$ 0.005

An area of great potential for monoclonal antibodies is the treatment of renal allograft rejection. Cosimi et al. reported the successful reversal of clinically demonstrated immunological rejection with the sole use of anti-T cell antibodies (17,30). A randomized trial of rejection treatment with OKT3 is currently being conducted in North America. The initial results show that the in vivo administration of monoclonal antibodies is reasonably well tolerated, although side effects, such as chills, tremors, and bronchospasms were observed. Endogenous mediators are set free through the process of cell opsonization, which explains the occurrence of some side effects as a "physiological response". Severe adverse reactions were observed occasionally in the form of pulmonary edema.

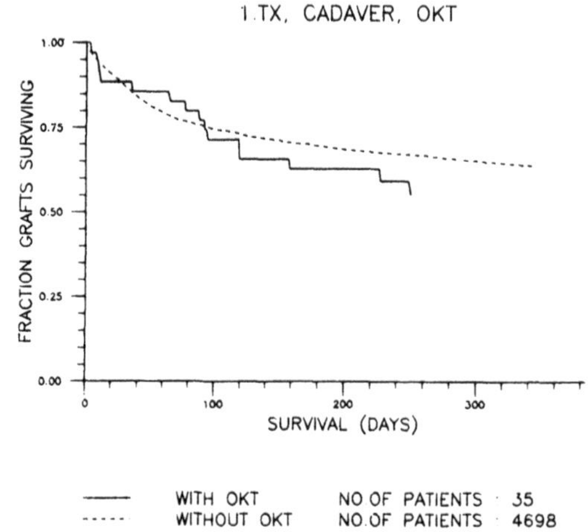

Figure 1. Actuarial graft survival rates of cadaver kidney transplants. The solid curve represents 35 patients treated for rejection with OKT3 monoclonal antibodies. The dotted line is the survival curve for grafts without monoclonal antibody treatment. There is no statistically significant difference between the two curves. All transplants were performed in 1982 and 1983. Data from the international Collaborative Transplant Study.

Monoclonal anti-T cell antibodies have proven extremely effective in reversing rejection, even in cases of steroid resistance. The T cells virtually disappear from the patient's circulation within minutes of antibody administration and the patient improves clinically. However, long-term graft survival does not appear to be improved significantly. Figure 1 shows us preliminary data in OKT3 treated patients transplanted at 5 different transplant centres. Their graft survival was not significantly different from that in conventionally treated patients. The data were derived from the Collaborative Transplant Study, an international collaborative effort of some 200 transplant centres in 24 countries.

What are the problems with monoclonal antibody treatment of rejection? Perhaps the most significant one is the fact that all patients who were treated developed antibodies against mouse immunoglobulin. Thus, monoclonal antibodies can be used for the treatment of a single rejection only; subsequent rejections must be treated with conventional immunosuppression. Since most patients go on to reject again, eventual graft outcome is not improved significantly. Currently, attempts are being made to induce tolerance to mouse immunoglobuline in order to make the administration of repeated courses of monoclonal antibodies possible.

Another difficulty with monoclonal antibody treatment was uncovered by Bach et al. (31). When patients are treated with OKT3 antibody, lymphocytes of the OKT3 phenotype and also those carrying the OKT4 or OKT8 phenotypes are removed from the patient's circulation. OKT3 cells remain absent for several days. However, cells expressing the OKT4 or OKT8 markers reappear within hours. Thus, antigenic modulation occurs in OKT3 treated patients, leading to the occurrence of cells carrying a new phenotype. Because the cells do not carry the OKT3 marker, subsequent administration of OKT3 antibody cannot affect them. This is another reason why the prophylactic use of monoclonal antibodies for prevention of graft rejection is impractical (32).

Recently, an antibody reactive against blast cells (CBL1) was used successfully for the treatment of kidney graft rejection in Japan (33). Although anti-T cell antibodies are equally effective, treatment with anti-blast cell antibody shows some interesting features. In contrast to OKT3, CBL1 does not cause any adverse side reactions. Moreover, the peripheral lymphocyte count is not affected. Thus, without depletion of lymphocytes, rejection is reversed. The authors interpret their results as indicating specific reactivity of CBL1 against immunoreactive cells attacking the graft, which represent only a small, barely noticeable fraction of the entire lymphocyte pool. They go on to speculate that depletion of the specific clone that reacts against the graft may eliminate subsequent rejections and thus make the repeated administration of antibody unnecessary. If borne out in further studies, this may indeed represent the long awaited breakthrough in rejection management.

To summarize, the use of monoclonal antibodies had led to impressive advances in clinical organ transplantation. The improved ability to measure immunological reactions by monitoring lymphocyte subpopulations, the reduction in GvHD through the elimination of T cells from bone marrow in vitro, and the in vivo treatment of renal allograft rejection, all have been demonstrated to be clinically effective. Whether overall improvements in transplant results can be achieved with these techniques remains to be shown. As with many new developments, the successful transition from use at a few expert centres to a broadbased utilization may prove to be difficult. Cost is another factor that is becoming increasingly important in medical care, even in special fields such as organ transplantation. Nevertheless, it can be easily predicted that further advances will follow rapidly and that monoclonal antibodies will play an important role in the future of clinical transplantation.

REFERENCES

1. Köhler G, Milstein C. Continuous cultures of fused cells secreting antibody of predefined specificity. Nature 1975;256:495–7.
2. Foster CS. Lymphocyte hybridomas. Cancer Treat Rev 1982;9:59–84.
3. Sharp TG, Sachs DH, Fauci AS, Messerschmidt GL, Rosenberg SA. T cell depletion of human bone marrow using monoclonal antibody and complement-mediated lysis. Transplantation 1983;35:112–20.
4. Friedrich W, O'Reilly RJ, Koziner B, Gebhard DF, Good RA, Evans RL. T-lymphocyte reconstitution in recipients of bone marrow transplants with and without GvHD. Blood 1982;59:696–701.
5. Atkinson K, Hansen JA, Storb R, Goehle S, Goldstein G, Thomas ED. T-cell subpopulations identified by monoclonal antibodies after human bone marrow transplantation. Blood 1982;59:1292–8.
6. Fox R, McMillan R, Spruce W, et al. Analysis of T lymphocytes after bone marrow transplantation using monoclonal antibodies. Blood 1982;60: 578–82.
7. Schroff RW, Gale RP, Fahey JL. Regeneration of T cell subpopulations after bone marrow transplantation. J Immunol 1982;129:1926–30.

8. Martin PJ, Shulman HM, Schubach WH, et al. Fatal EBV-associated proliferation of donor B cells following treatment of acute graft-versus-host disease with a murine monoclonal anti-T cell antibody. N Engl J Med (in press).
9. Müller-Ruchholtz W, Wottge HU, Müller-Hermelink HK. Bone marrow transplantation in rats across strong histocompatibility barriers by selective elimination of lymphoid cells in donor marrow. Transplant Proc 1976;8:537–40.
10. Thierfelder S, Hoffmann-Fezer G, Rodt H, Doxiadis I, Eulitz M, Kummer U. Antilymphocytic antibodies in marrow transplantation. Transplantation 1983;35:249–54.
11. Vallera DA, Soderling CCB, Kersey JH. Bone marrow transplantation across major histocompatibility barriers in mice. J Immunol 1982;128: 871–5.
12. Prentice HG, Blacklock HA, Janossy G, et al. Use of anti-T-cell monoclonal antibody OKT3 to prevent acute graft-versus-host disease in allogeneic bone-marrow transplantation for acute leukaemia. Lancet 1982;i:700–3.
13. Filipovich A, McGlave PB, Ramsay NK, Goldstein G, Warkentin PI, Kersey JH. Pretreatment of donor bone marrow with monoclonal antibody OKT3 for prevention of acute graft-versus-host disease in allogeneic histocompatible bone-marrow transplantation. Lancet 1982;i: 1266–9.
14. Hayward AR, Murphy S, Githens J, Troup G, Ambruso D. Failure of a pan-reactive anti-T cell antibody, OKT3, to prevent graft versus host disease in severe combined immunodeficiency. J Pediatr 1982;100:665–8.
15. Medical News. Mismatches marrow grafts succeed thanks to two anti-T-cell agents. JAMA 1983;249:1687–9.
16. Ritz J, Sallan SE, Bast RC, et al. Autologous bone-marrow transplantation in CALLA-positive acute lymphoblastic leukaemia after in-vitro treatment with J5 monoclonal antibody and complement. Lancet 1982;ii: 60–3.
17. Cosimi AB, Colvin RB, Burton RC, et al. Use of monoclonal antibodies to T-cell subsets for immunologic monitoring and treatment in recipients of renal allografts. N Engl J Med 1981;305:308–14.
18. Ellis TM, Lee HM, Mohanakumar T. Alterations in human regulatory T lymphocyte subpopulations after renal allografting. J Immunol 1981;127: 2199–203.
19. Mazaheri R, Laupacis A, Keown P, Howson W, Sinclair NR, Stiller CR. Lymphocyte subsets in the allograft recipient. Transplant Proc 1982;14: 676–8.
20. Nanni-Costa A, Vangelista A, Frasca GM, Stefoni S, Bonomini V. T-cell subsets in renal allograft recipients. Transplant Proc 1983;15:1176–7.
21. Binkley WF, Valenzuela R, Braun WE, Deodhar SD, Novick AC, Steinmuller DR. Flow cytometry quantitation of peripheral blood T-cell subsets in human renal allograft recipients. Transplant Proc 1983;15:1163–5.
22. Carter NP, Cullen PR, Thompson JF, Bewick ALT, Wood RFM, Morris PJ. Monitoring lymphocyte subpopulations in renal allograft recipients. Transplant Proc 1983;15:1157–9.
23. Guttmann RD, Poulsen RS. Fluorescence activated cell sorter analysis of lymphocyte subsets after renal transplantation. Transplant Proc 1983; 15:1160–2.
24. Chatenoud L, Chkoff N, Kreis H, Bach JF. Interest in and limitations of monoclonal anti-T-cell antibodies for the follow-up of renal transplant

patients. Transplantation 1983;36:45–50.
25. Daniel V, Opelz G. Lymphocyte subset monitoring in renal transplant recipients. Transplant Proc (in press).
26. Colvin RB, Cosimi AB, Burton RC, et al. Circulating T-cell subsets in 72 human renal allograft recipients. Transplant Proc 1983;15:1166–9.
27. Platt FL, LeBien TW, Michael AF. Interstitial mononuclear cell populations in renal graft rejection. J Exp Med 1982;155:17–30.
28. De Waele M, Thielemans C, Van Camp BKG. Characterization of immunoregulatory T cells in EBV-induced infectious mononucleosis by monoclonal antibodies. N Engl J Med 1981;304:460–2.
29. Schooley RT, Hirsch MS, Colvin RB, et al. Association of herpesvirus infection with T-lymphocyte subset alterations, glomerulopathy, and opportunistic infections after renal transplantation. N Engl J Med 1983; 308:307–13.
30. Cosimi AB, Burton RC, Colvin RB, et al. Treatment of acute renal allograft rejection with OKT3 monoclonal antibody. Transplantation 1981;32: 535–9.
31. Bach JF, Dardenne M, Chatenoud L. Immunomodulation of T cells by thymic hormone and monoclonal anti-T cell antibody. Transplant Proc 1982;14: 509–12.
32. Chatenoud L, Baudrihaye MF, Chkoff N, Kreis H, Bach JF. Immunologic follow-up of renal allograft recipients treated prophylactically by OKT3 alone. Transplant Proc 1983;15:643–5.
33. Takahashi H, Okazaki H, Terasaki PI, et al. Reversal of transplant rejection by monoclonal antiblast antibody. Lancet 1983;ii:1155–8.

DISCUSSION

Moderators: A.B. Glassman, B. Löwenberg

D.W. van Bekkum:

According to two groups in the United States, 70% of all the cases of chronic graft-versus-host disease were resulting from patients that already had suffered from acute graft-versus-host disease. So, 30% appears to be primary. I do not know whether this is a very slowly developing graft-versus-host disease, or that it is a new syndrome.

The second observation is that cyclosporin A, following allogeneic bone marrow transplantations, in the rat model is quite powerful in preventing graft-versus-host disease. If you stop the administration of cyclosporin A after four or five months, at the time when the non cyclosporin treated animals are already recovering – as far as they have survived – you will find that a large proportion of the cyclosporin A treated animals suddenly starts to develop a syndrome with mostly skin manifestations very similar to chronic graft-versus-host disease in human beings.

B. Löwenberg:

Dr. de Vries-Hospers, is it possible to replace amphoterycin B by giving ketaconazole?

H.G. de Vries-Hospers (Groningen, The Netherlands):

Ketaconazole is an imidazole antifungal agent which is partially absorbed from the gut after oral administration. The excretion of the drug into the saliva could be of advantage for suppression of yeasts in the oropharynx*. A few studies have been performed in immunocompromised patients in which ketoconazole was compared with a placebo**,***. Therapeutic efficacy of ketoconazole in oropharyngeal candidiasis could be demonstrated although it was less than desired. Meunier-Carpentier et al., studied the effect of nystatin and ketoconazole on orapharyngeal candidiasis; in the small number

* Brass C, Galgiani JN, Blaschke TF, Defelice R, O'Reilly RA, Stevens DA. Disposition of ketaconazole, an oral antifungal, in humans. Antimicrob Agents Chemotherapy 1982;21:151–8.
** Brincker H. Prevention of mycosis in granulocytopenic patients with pro: phylactic ketonazole treatment. Mykosen 1983;26:242–7.
*** Hughes WT, Bartley DL, Patterson GG, Tufenkeji H. Ketoconazole and candidiasis: a controlled study. J Inf Dis 1983;147:1060–3.

of so-treated patients nystatin was somewhat more effective*. Hann et al., compared a combination of nystatin and amphotericin B with ketoconazole alone and found the latter to be superior, except in patients who received allogeneic bone-marrow transplantation**. This could be explained by the lower serum levels of ketoconazole in transplanted patients. In the University Hospital of Groningen ketoconazole was given to a small number of leukemic patients during chemotherapy. Subsequently serum levels were measured. These serum levels were found to be lower than in normal subjects after the same dosages. In patients in whom the absorption from the GI-tract is uncertain, the effect of ketoconazole in the oropharynx is also uncertain.

B. Löwenberg:

Dr. de Vries-Hospers, you compared selective decontamination with controls. You had successful SD patients and non-successful SD patients. How did you analyse non-successfully decontaminated patients in the SD group.

H.G. de Vries-Hospers:

All patients were free of Gram-negatives.

B. Löwenberg:

So, they all were successful?

H.G. de Vries-Hospers:

Occasionally cultures were positive. However, if we found resistant bacteria, we changed the SD-regimen.

B. Löwenberg:

A second question is: Many of our patients with leukemia had to receive systemic antibiotics. The data you showed were the net result of SD treatment plus systemic antibodies, which may have interfered with the GI flora. How did this interfere?

H.G. de Vries-Hospers:

This is difficult, but usually in the trial period we use gentamycin, ampicillin and ticarcillin for systemic treatment, and especially ticarcillin may disturb the GI-flora. Sometimes we could see that the enterococci decreased in concentration, but we never did see an overgrowth by resistant Gram-negative rods, which could be expected. This is why, particularly during

* Meunier-Carpentier F, Snoeck R, Ceuppens AM, Klastersky J. Treatment of oropharyngeal candidiasis in cancer patients. In: Proceedings of the 13th International Congress of Chemotherapy, part 40. Antifungal therapy with ketoconazole. Vienna 1983.
** Hann IN, Corringham R, Keanny M, et al. Ketoconazole versus nystatin plus amphotericin B for fungal prophylaxis in severely immunocompromised patients. Lancet 1982;i:826–9

systemic treatment, selective decontamination must be continued to compensate for the decrease of the colonisation resistance which may occur during systemic treatment.

B. Löwenberg:

Did systemic treatment not influence the results in any way?

H.G. de Vries-Hospers:

Sofar, no.

J.P. Hester (Houston, USA):

Dr. Ho, if you doubled the dose, is there an explanation for why you did not get twice the plasma concentration in the patients?

W.G. Ho:

That is an interesting question, to which I really have no answer. I do not think that at this point, we have really gone into the finer points of understanding what is going on when we administer either the immune plasma or the immunoglobulins. We were happy at this point to see some clinical effect on the CMV infections. It is only now that we are trying to answer some of those questions. I would be glad to make a note of that question and add it to our list of interesting things that have yet to be answered.

B. Löwenberg:

In Rotterdam we are infusing patients with an immunoglobulin preparation also with a high CMV titer. We found quite some variation in the kinetics of these CMV titers from patient to patient. As far as the failures are concerned, did you monitor as to whether you achieved an effective titer in those patients until the next transfusion?

W.G. Ho:

Yes. The titer levels are monitored in every patient, and not only by one method. We are currently carrying out a complement fixation test, radioimmuno assay and ELISA on every patient. There is some variation from patient to patient, from week to week, as the infusion is given. However, the trend is about the same: An immediate rise, a quick fall within the first 24 hours and a levelling off in a week's period to a level that we feel is acceptable.

W.G. Ho:

Dr. Hester, you are sure there are data to suggest that the presence of hemorrhage is an adverse factor in the induction of remission in leukemic patients? How do you define hemorrhage? There is hemorrhage and hemorrhage: You can have petechiae, you can have echymosis, you can have hematuria, you can have epistaxis or massive hemorrhage. What is hemorrhage in that respect?

J.P. Hester:

Dr. Ho, we do not consider petechiae to constitute major hemorrhage. Major hemorrhage is defined in our unit as CNS hemorrhage, pulmonary hemorrhage, and gastrointestinal hemorrhage which cannot be controlled. Hematuria, gingival bleeding, petechiae, epistaxis are not considered to be major, and they do not usually result in the death of the patient.

A.B. Glassman:

I would like to ask Dr. Schooley and Dr. Ho to respons to the following question: You have demonstrated that there is a reduction in clinical CMV-infection severity. One, by the use of immunoglobulin, and the other by the use of interferon. What about a synergistic effect of using both at the same time? Or are you entering through the same mechanism of host response by the use of the immunoglobulin and the interferon?

R.T. Schooley (Boston, USA):

I think that is an excellent question. We obviously have not looked at the two together. I would hope that they are operating through different mechanisms. Eventually, as we get more of a feel for the toxicity and efficacy of these single agents, we are going to do some more innovative things like combining different approaches.

W.G. Ho:

I think I have very little to add to that comment. It is only now that we are realising that there is something that seems to make a difference in CMV infections. We are trying to accumulate data in order to study more scientifically what is going on here. But a combination might be useful.

A.B. Glassman:

Dr. de Vries-Hospers, when I visited the University Hospital in Groningen, I was impressed by the fact that the major trauma patients are also on a prophylactic antibiotic protocol that is given orally in a paste. It is colistin, fungisone and tobramycin. I was not convinced that there was a lot of data as to the emergence of resistant organisms. Although you mentioned in a rather casual way that one just changes the antibiotic, are we producing super-strains of resistant organisms?

H.G. de Vries-Hospers:

Sometimes we do isolate resistant strains, but we change the SD regimen as soon as we find resistant bacteria. This in general results in disappearance of resistant bacteria before they can cause problems. We have, however, had a problem with a resistant Serratia-species which was resistant to all drugs available for selective decontamination at that time. But this was one case in seven years.

M. Hébert (Quebec, Canada):

Dr. de Vries-Hospers, in the study that you presented, you use a lot of antibiotics. I would like to comment on whether you observe any kind of side-effects with those antibiotics, which would force you to perhaps withdraw some of your patients from your study?

H.G. de Vries-Hospers:

Polymyxin in general causes less side effects. Some patients become nauseous, but then we can change over to one of the other drugs. Co-trimoxazole may give skin rashes or other allergic reactions. The same is true for nalidixic acid, which also may induce nausea. Often it is difficult to say what the reason is for the nausea, because all patients are also treated with cytostatic drugs. However, in general it is no problem for the patient to take the drugs. As the fecal cultures become and remain free of Gram-negatives, we have a check whether the patients really ingest these drugs in a sufficient dose.

K. Sintnicolaas (Rotterdam, The Netherlands):

Dr. Hester, you presented data comparing the random single donor platelets and multiple donor platelets, with better results, I believe, for random single donor platelets. We have conducted a study, where we also compared random single donor platelets and multiple donor platelets. We randomized the patients and gave them exactly the same number of platelets per transfusion. After transfusion we measured platelet increments and calculated the recoveries. We found better recoveries for the single donor platelets*.

I have some questions about your study: I wonder how you select the patients for random single donor platelets or for multiple donor platelets. Did you measure the post-transfusion platelet recoveries and did you find differences between the groups? Could you detect platelet antibodies in the patients and were there also differences between the groups?

J.P. Hester:

The data you saw about single donor and multiple random donors was a study from 1980 to 1982. Since 1982, 80–90% of our patients receive single donor fresh concentrates, rather than multiple random. There are two reasons: I think that of all the parameters which influence transfusion, alloimmunization may emerge to be the most important aspect of the transfusion. We find that supporting patients with a limited number of donors allows us to transfuse some patients up to nine months. When we have patients who are alloimmunized to random pooled platelets, I have very little way of finding a matched HLA donor.

Additionally, we have done platelet function studies on random pooled units which often represent a mixture of fresh to 72 hour stored concentrates. In general, pooled random platelets, when they have aged, do not

* Sintnicolaas K, Vriesendorp HM, Sizoo W, et al. Delayed alloimmunisation by random single donor platelet transfusions. A randomized study to compare single donor and multiple donor platelet transfusions in cancer patients with severe thrombocytopenia. Lancet 1981;i:750–4.

give us three days of hemostasis, although there is a transient period of circulation in peripheral blood post-transfusion. If hemostasis cannot be achieved with stored platelets in a manner comparable to fresh platelets, then we would feel that the use of stored platelets would not cost effective nor physiologically be appropriate for the patient.

K. Sintnicolaas:

To be specific, can you give the frequencies of alloimmunization in both groups of patients? How much is the reduction?

J.P. Hester:

Alloimmunization is defined in my unit, as less than 10% post-transfusion recovery, in the absence of pneumonia or septicaemia, or active hemorrhage. I find that at least 80% of our patients, if they are transfused long enough will become immunized to a modest degree or to a severe degree.

K. Sintnicolaas:

But do you not have the comparative figures for single donors and multiple donors?

J.P. Hester:

No. As I said, to sort out immunization from all the other variables you need a model that will tell you what percentage of the recovery is affected by hemorrhage, what percentage of the recovery is affected by sepsis. Then we could distinguish between single donor versus random pool. I do not have an answer for that at this time.

B. Löwenberg:

A question which is somewhat related to the last question: I think you made the statement that the beautiful platelet survival curves which one finds in normal patients cannot be demonstrated in patients with leukemia, even if they are not clearly alloimmunized or have splenomegaly, or for some other apparent reason. Do you have any idea of what factors may be involved in this phenomenon? Any reason why they have different, shortened survivals?

J.P. Hester:

We have patients who have never been transfused with any blood products, who are a-splenic from surgery, and who fail to get any post-transfusion increment and in whom transfused platelets did not circulate. I suspect there must be some naturally occurring antibodies to platelets, but I have no scientific to support it.

May I ask a question? Does Dr. Persijn have an explanation for why the transplant patients do better with multiple blood transfusions?

G.G. Persijn (Leiden, The Netherlands):

Well, the mechanism of how blood transfusion works is very speculative and it will take a long time to clarify that. It might be due to enhancing antibodies or suppressor cells or maybe a combination of mechanisms*, we really do not know.

W.G. Ho:

Dr. Hester, first of all I want to congratulate you on your efforts in trying to sort out what is sense and what is nonsense in regard to this type of therapy. There is another model that is being used by the Seattle Group. (Dr. Slichter**), which involves thrombocytopenic dogs. In that situation Dr. Slichter tries to determine what dose of platelets might effect the level and what are actual indications for administering platelets. She uses as donors DLA identical matches, actually syngeneic matches for the dogs, as well as non-related donors. The fact that she does see an effect of DLA matching in that respect means that she sees as well a dose relation with regard to the development of alloimmunization, although the exact dose relation is not clear. Most of the dogs that received 4 transfusions or a greater number will develop alloimmunization, although there are some dogs that you can keep transfusing from various and unrelated sources who will never become immunized, as you will also see a few who will become immunized after one single transfusion.
As a point to determine when to give a transfusion, she is using $10x10^9/l$ as the cut-off point, based on the presence of blood in the stools of these dogs.

A.B. Glassman:

I would like to make one more comment. Not all of the disappearance of platelets may be on an immunologic basis. We know that some of the patients with a variety of myeloproliferative disorders have aberrations of the prostaglandin and arachadonic acid metabolism, and this obviously can activate the platelets. When one injects platelets, it takes one to two hours within the intravascular space to adapt so that they can circulate at an optimal level. I think that some of the reasons that we do not see an added increment in some of the patients with myeloproliferative disorders are on a non-immunologic basis, probably because of biochemical function and metabolic impairment. Not everything is immunology, we can still have some general thoughts.

J.M. Middeldorp (Groningen, The Netherlands):

Does Dr. Ho have experience with plasma or immunoglobulin preparations from normal seropositive donors? Secondly, does Dr. Ho have experience in the use of plasma in the treatment of acute CMV-infection?

* Singal DP, Joseph S, Szewczuk MR. Possible mechanisms of the beneficial effect of pretransplant blood transfusion on renal allograft survival in man. Transplant Proc 1982;XIV:316–8.

** Slichter SJ. Controversies in platelet transfusion therapy. Ann Res Med 1980;31:509–40.

W.G. Ho:

In regards to your first question, I have to say "No". The only immunoglobulin that we have been using so far has been provided by the Cutter Laboratories. Now that we have some data that the immunoglobulin is useful, we are still concerned that there may not be a widespread application of the immunoglobulin. The financial considerations are horrendous. It is estimated that a dose of 20 cc per kilogram per week for 20 weeks comes to $ 2,000 per week per patients. That is not something we can give every patient. There are other preparations made available with a hyperimmune-specific CMV-globulin which will be used in a much smaller dose. But we did not use any other preparation at this point.

With regard to the actual treatment of established CMV-infections with either plasma or immunoglobulin, we have not done that because our protocol has been to try to prevent in the first place. We are discouraged by the fact that there was actually no reduction in the incidence, so that the patients who were actually receiving immunoglobulin did develop CMV-infections. We did continue the administration of the plasma or the immunoglobulin. We did not see any effect at that point. It is similar to the situation that one gets with the treatment of specific anti-viral agents, chemotherapeutics or biological modifyers. Once the infection is established, there is no effect.

R. Schweitzer (Frankfurt, FRG):

So far, we got first results from the department of pediatrics. University of Frankfurt am Main. Children suffering from acute leukemia could be protected from CMV-infection when treated prophylactically with our CMV-immunoglobulin. Now a multicentre trial will be arranged to administer this immunoglobulin prophylactically for all children suffering from acute myeloid leukemia.

J.M. Middeldorp:

Your immune preparation is prepared from randomly selected sero-positive donors?

R. Schweitzer:

Yes, it is.

W.G. Ho:

Our selection criteria are those patients who actually are positive only at the very low level. That is essentially sero-negative, by the CMV-trials that we have been doing. We are not choosing seropositive, it is seronegative and the titers for the immune plasma were 1 to 16 or less. Not all of them become negative as we go along. What we have found is that some of those have a level of 1 to 32. This was based on some data that the Seattle Group had on a larger group of patients*. Some of those patients, actually,

* Meyers JD, Flournoy N, Thomas ED. Nonbacterial pneumonia after allogeneic marrow transplantation; A review of ten years experience. Rev Infect Dis 1982;4:1119–32.

were not protected from their infections, so we actually included them. We are not trying to separate exogenous from endogenous in this situation.

A.B. Glassman:

Dr. Opelz, in your very excellent review and in the predictions for the future, you have talked so far only about monoclonal antibodies made in species other than man. It is my understanding that there are some hybridomas of man. Do you see some future for that in immunemodulation and transplantation?

G. Opelz:

I certainly do see a future. It is a matter of time. The discouraging thing is that the monoclonals that are produced with human cell lines so far have not turned out to be sufficiently potent or sustainable so that one could really use them, certainly not in the clinic.

J.P. Hester:

Dr. Opelz, in some of the patients you have seen chills. Did you see changes in leukocyte counts and platelets after the administration or infusion of these antibodies? The reason for my question is: Patients who are routinely getting leukocyte interferon in our hospital develop chills, fever, a leukopenia and a drop in platelet count as a biological indicator of responsivity. Since these are animal-derived materials, are you seeing a similar sing?

G. Opelz:

There is no consistency, it is not predictable and it is very variable. You will see severe thrombocytopenia in some patients, but only in a few. There is no way of telling ahead of time what will happen.

III. ORGAN PRESERVATION

ORGANIZATION AND EFFECTIVENESS IN DONOR PROCUREMENT AND TRANSPLANTATION

R.J. Ploeg

INTRODUCTION

Over the past decades renal transplantation has been transformed from an experimental clinical procedure to an established method of treatment of end-stage renal disease (ESRD). From 1975 through 1982 the number of patients suffering from end-stage renal disease doubled in several european countries (Figure 1). According to the registry report at the London Meeting of the European Dialysis and Transplantation Association (EDTA) in 1982, 65,386 patients were treated in Europe with hemodialysis, 6,092 patients with peritoneal dialysis, and 15,318 patients did have a functioning graft (1).

In The Netherlands e.g., the incidence of end-stage renal disease per million population was 25 in 1975 and 42 in 1980. It has been calculated that the incidence will have increased to 60 new patients with ESRD per million population per year in 1990.

Treatment of end-stage renal disease is life saving but expensive. However, it is well known that by increasing the transplantation activity the total costs of the ESRD-budget will decrease, whereas more years of life and, especially, a higher quality of life are gained (2,3,4).

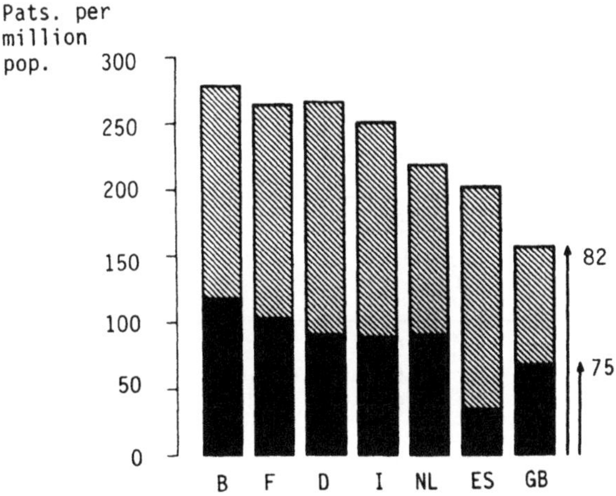

Figure 1. Number of ESRD – patients in 7 European countries according to the EDTA – registry report 1983.

Currently the majority of transplantations in Europe has to be performed with cadaveric donor organs, whereas only small numbers of patients can be transplanted with a kidney from a living related donor. This dependence of cadaveric donor organs reveals a major problem in organ transplantation: donor shortage. With greater reliance on cadaveric grafts for treatment of patients with end-stage renal disease, and the advent of hepatic, cardiac and pancreatic transplantation, an increased number of cadaveric organs must inevitably be required. It is one of the main tasks of the organ sharing services to cope with these problems.

ORGAN SHARING AND EUROTRANSPLANT

Currently several organ sharing services are operating through Europe on a national or international basis, involving numerous dialysis centres, tissue-typing laboratories and transplant centres. These organizations are called France-, U.K.-, Scandia-, Inter-, Italy- and Eurotransplant.

The idea to start the Eurotransplant organization dates back to 1967 and was proposed by Prof. Dr. J.J. van Rood. The need for a large donor and recipient pool was strongly felt in order to achieve the aim of finding, within the enormous polymorphism of the HLA-system, optimaly matched donor-recipient combinations. Such optimaly matched combinations were taken to be mandatory for improving kidney graft survival, as illustrated by the results of identical sibling transplantation. The main objectives of the Eurotransplant organization are:

- to maximize the survival time of transplanted organs through tissue-typing and matching,
- to create a structure, in which as many patients as possible will receive an appropriate organ as soon as possible,
- to obtain, by the creation of an efficient administrative structure, a high utilisation rate of available organs.

To achieve these aims, the organization established a network of laboratories for donor- and recipient typing and cross-matching purposes. Standardized techniques and reagents were introduced. A central registration of all potential recipients within Eurotransplant was built up, is daily updated

Table I. Number of collaborating centres in Eurotransplant and number of patients on the waiting list per country.

Country	Typing centres	Transplant centres	Number of patients on waiting list	
			1981	1982
Austria	4	4	313	358
Belgium	6	6	316	394
Germany	24	20	1781	2128
Luxemburg	1	1	-	12
The Netherlands	6	7	525	650
Others	-	-	234	214
Total	41	38	3169	3756

and supplies a regular feed-back of information. In addition a system of selection procedures was accomplished that functions with the shortest delay and the least effort. A very essential part of the organization was formed by the creation of a communication centre with expertise in organizational aspects of donor procurement, organ transplantation, transportation and financing.

The number of tissue-typing laboratories, transplant centres and number of kidney patients waiting for a transplant in 1982 per collaborating country are shown in Table I. All relevant data of the patients on the waiting list are centrally stored in the Eurotransplant computer in Leiden. With this computer not only selection procedures are performed, when a donor becomes available, but also follow-up analyses of transplanted patients can be carried out.

Whenever a potential donor becomes available, the blood group and HLA-type will be investigated by one of the participating tissue-typing laboratories. With the results of these tests a selection procedure can be started by means of a telex connection with the central computer. The selection criteria are ABO- and HLA-compatibility as well as the clinical urgency and the time on dialysis. Within Eurotransplant, donor-recipient combinations are matched according to a combined HLA- A+B/DR scheme. Highest priority is given to AB/DR-identical combinations, followed by DR identical/one AB-mismatch and AB-identical/one DR mismatch combinations, and so forth. Although some of the kidneys are used in the centre where they were retrieved, the fast majority of donor kidneys (80%) are transferred to another transplant centre. This exchange policy is reflected in improved matching rates (5).

In 1982 the Eurotransplant waiting list increased from 3,196 to 3,765 (+ 19%). In the same year 1,038 cadaveric donors were reported; 812 donors were nephrectomized, out of whom 1,493 kidneys could be transplanted. At the end of 1983 the number of patients on the waiting list had increased to 4,319. Currently the mean waiting time within the Eurotransplant system is 27 months, whereas the medium waiting time is only 16 months. This difference can be explained by an increasing number of highly sensitized potential recipients, who have to wait several years before they are actually transplanted.

DONOR PROCUREMENT

In spite of the tremendous efforts of all organ sharing services, including Eurotransplant, all transplant waiting lists have increased since the number of retrieved donor kidneys could not meet the demand of recipients waiting

Table II. Kidneys available per million inhabitants – ET 1982.

Country	Population (in mill.)	Kidneys available	Per million inhabitants
Austria	7.5	141	18.8
Belgium	9.9	139	14.0
Germany	61,6	812	13.2
The Netherlands	14.3	313	21.9

for a suitable organ. The donor procurement activities in various countries participating within Eurotransplant are shown in Table II. In a combined effort of the National Bureau of Health Statistics and Eurotransplant, an attempt was made to estimate retrospectivily the number of potential organ donors per year in The Netherlands. The number of patients who died of causes not interfering with potential donorship and who were not identified as being suitable organ donors from a technical point of view, was found to be approximately 830 in 1978. In order to investigate the factors which were responsible for this discrepancy in the numbers of actually identified and possibly suitable organ donors, a questionnaire was sent to 181 hospitals throughout the country. Of the 101 hospitals that responded, none objected to the idea of performing donor nephrectomies on the basis of ethical or other principal reasons. In fact, in 43% of these hospitals donor nephrectomies had been performed at least once. A reluctant attitude towards active co-operation in donor referral was found to be mainly due to the fact that the complete donor procedure is usually time-consuming, and disturbes the daily routine within the hospital. Especially, the task of obtaining the formal consent from the relatives appeared to reduce the motivation of the hospital staff to initiate a donor procedure. From the results of these inquiries it was concluded that the shortage of suitable organ donors in The Netherlands was not primarily caused by an absolute shortage of organ donors, but, instead, by a shortage in the number of potential donor identifications and referrals (6,7). Thus, apart from the persisting need of providing educational information to the public continuously, the main challenge was felt to be formed by the need of stimulating the medical profession into a higher state of active alertness concerning organ procurement. For that purpose the provision of professional education as well as offering active assistance was thought to be mandatory.

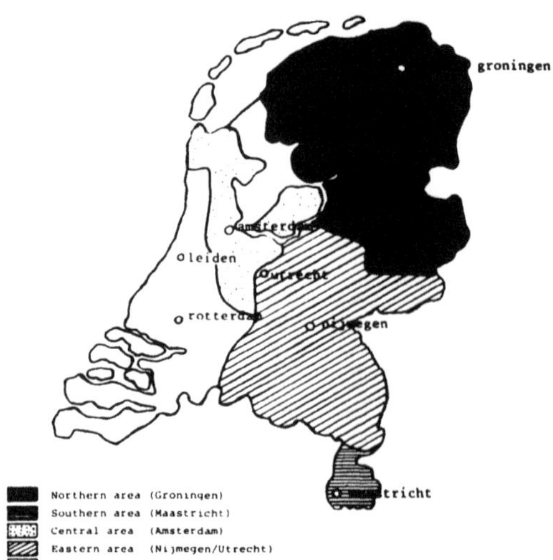

Figure 2. Transplant co-ordination areas in The Netherlands.

TRANSPLANT CO-ORDINATORS

In order to accomplish a satisfactory increase in the number of organ donations five transplant co-ordinators were appointed in The Netherlands. As it was felt that a more efficient and effective approach towards all possible target groups, eventually participating in donor procurements, was necessary, The Netherlands were divided into five geographical areas (8). These five co-ordination areas, each with a known number of potential donor hospitals, could be approached by the individual co-ordinator. Vice versa the hospitals themselves learned to know exactly whom to contact for advice and practical help in case of a donor procedure (Figure 2).

ORGANIZATION WITHIN A CO-ORDINATION AREA

The potential donor hospitals were left completely free as how to use the services of the regional transplant co-ordinator. Thus, several options concerning the organizational participation of the transplant co-ordinator were offered to each hospital. These options ranged from a 100% involvement in every donor procedure on the one hand to no involvement at all on the other, which latter option implied a completely self-reliant effectuation of every donor procedure by the hospital itself. Alternative options and modifications were introduced by the transplant co-ordinator to the medical and nursing staff of each hospital, and amply discussed. On the basis of this information a working agreement between the hospital and the transplant co-ordinator was achieved, according to the specific needs and demands of each individual hospital. In addition every co-ordinator distributed his regional protocol containing the logistics of a donor procedure and the essentials in donor management. To facilitate organ retrieval within a certain donor area the surgeons of the various transplant teams offered, if required, the service of a "mobile nefrectomy team". In case the local donor hospital would not be able to perform the donor operation itself the appropriate transplant centre would provide a team to retrieve and preserve the organs. The hospital staffs were asked to contact the regional transplant co-ordinator as soon as organ donation was considered. This allows the co-ordinator to get involved at an early stage in the process of an organ donation and to proceed to the local donor hospital in order to judge the suitability of a donor according to the current clinical criteria. If appropriate the co-ordinator accepts the donor and the donor procedure is started. Concerning the brain death criteria the co-ordinator looks after the completion of brain stem examinations and additional informative tests like the EEG and a carotic angiography. Advice and help on medical, organizational and legal aspects are offered. If required the co-ordinator takes over the treatment of the donor in order to allow the referring doctor to continue his daily work. If requested, the co-ordinator asks his mobile nefrectomy team to come to the hospital. In case the house surgeon is perfectly capable of performing the donor operation himself, the transplant co-ordinator assists the local surgeon, preserves the organs and prepares them for transportation in a standard way. The co-ordinator as well as the mobile nefrectomy team are permanently available and provide a 24 hours service, 7 days a week.

PRESENT STATUS OF DONOR PROCUREMENT IN THE NETHERLANDS

From 1975 until 1980 the number of referrals in The Netherlands seemed to have reached a plateau (9). During this period an average number of 187 organ donors was reported anually. 1981 showed a considerable increase in the number of donor referrals: 250 organ donors were reported, an increase of 36% since 1980. A total of 160 donors was actually nephrectomized out of whom 316 kidneys could be used for transplantation. These numbers remained stable in 1982, whereas another increase could be seen in 1983, since 345 kidneys could be offered to the Eurotransplant pool and subsequently be transplanted. Concerning multi organ procurement an increasing number of "other organs" and transplantable tissues were referred and actually retrieved over the last years. Mainly liver, heart, cornea and skin. Within his/her area the co-ordinator tries to stimulate hospital staffs to ask consent from the relatives for organ donation in general instead of for kidney donation only.

By this time almost all potential donor hospitals in each Dutch co-ordination area have been contacted. Professional education on organ donation as well as on transplantation has been given to medical and nursing staffs. Currently most hospitals are quite happy to co-operate with their regional co-ordinator, thus avoiding the time consuming and laborious accomplishment of a donor procedure. Many doctors in charge of a donor call the co-ordinator at an early stage as soon as an organ donation is considered. It is too early to conclude that the increase over the last three years in the number of donor referrals and actually nephrectomized kidneys is caused by the five transplant co-ordinators. However, one could suggest that the establishment of transplant co-ordination in The Netherlands has contributed to a higher state of active alertness in our donor hospitals.

CONCLUSIONS

In conclusion, a dramatic increase of ESRD-patients in Europe over the past 5 years has resulted in an enormous waiting list for transplantation.

In spite of the tremendous efforts of the organ sharing services the number of retrieved donor kidneys could not meet the demands of recipients waiting for a suitable and well-matched organ. Thus, there seems to persist a continuing need for a large international donor-recipient pool. The permanent shortage of donor organs reveals a major problem in transplantation: the dependence on cadaveric donor organs. However, this situation might be paradoxal: a shortage in the face of plenty, since there is no absolute shortage of organ donors, but, instead, a shortage of donor referrals. Therefore the medical profession has to be stimulated towards active donor procurement.

The organ sharing services and the transplant co-ordinators positively influence the organization and effectiveness of donor procurement and transplantation.

ACKNOWLEDGEMENT

The author is indebted to Ms. Mariëlle Boesten for preparing the manuscript and to the staff of the Eurotransplant Foundation for supplying the information on which this paper is based.

REFERENCES

1. Proceedings of the European Dialysis and Transplantation Association. London, 1983, Pitman, Vol. 20:5–12.
2. Lowrie EG, Hampers CL. The success of Medicare's end-stage renal disease program. N Engl J Med 1981;305:434–8.
3. Iglehart JK. Funding the end-stage renal disease program. N Engl J Med 1982;306:492–6.
4. De By TMMH, D'Amaro JD, Persijn GG, Barneveld-Binkhuyzen FH, Cohen B. A retrospective analysis of hospital haemodialysis and kidney transplantation costs in The Netherlands. Neth J Med 1982;25:83–7.
5. Eurotransplant Annual Report 1982. Persijn GG, Hendriks F, Cohen B, eds. Leiden, 1982.
6. Bart KJ, Macon EJ, Whittier FC, Baldwin RJ, Blount JH. Increasing the supply of cadaveric kidneys for transplantation. Transplantation 1981; 31:383–7.
7. Bart KJ, Macon EJ, Whittier FC, Baldwin RJ, Blount JH. Cadaveric kidneys for transplantation. Transplantation 1981;31:379–82.
8. Ploeg RJ. The Dutch view on transplant co-ordination. Proceedings EDTA-EDTNA, Madrid 1982;10:106–12.
9. Eurotransplant Annual Reports 1975–1981. Cohen B, ed. Leiden: Eurotransplant Foundation.

ORGANISATION OF A HOSPITAL BONE MARROW PANEL

D.C.O. James

INTRODUCTION

The first unrelated bone marrow transplant carried out in 1973 at Westminster Hospital was possible only after considerable effort in locating the compatible donor (1). It was obvious that a panel or register of previous HLA-tested donors based on the blood transfusion service system was highly desirable. Because of financial restraints, the register was not commenced until 1975, but since then a steady input of about 5000 names yearly has been possible and the initial target of 50,000 has been exceeded.

All the donors have volunteered specifically to give bone marrow, and also other blood products but for use only of bone marrow transplant (BMTp) patients. All are fully informed before donation that bone marrow (BM) donation requires the use of general anesthesia and an overnight stay in hospital.

Origins and progress of the register

Although BMTp is now a recognized effective treatment for immune deficiency, aplastic anemia, acute leukemias, inborn errors of metabolism, B thalassemias etc., its use has in the main been restricted to patients with compatible sibling donors. Since the chance of finding a compatible sibling within a family is only 1 in 4, the majority of patients with bone marrow disease cannot receive a transplant unless a compatible donor can be found from outside the family.

The successful grafting of bone marrow from an unrelated donor into a child with chronic granulomatous disease was carried out at Westminster Hospital, London in 1973. However, the finding of the donor was not achieved without considerable effort, including appeals to the public using press, radio and television. These resulted in massive short-term responses from the public which disrupted hospital telephonic communications etc. and indicated the need for the setting up of a bone marrow donor register with a planned recruiting and HLA-testing programme. Adequate funds only became available for this project in 1974 with the need to search for a donor for a child with Wiskott-Aldridge syndrome, the fund-raising initially being inspired by the child's mother.

The many problems of donor recruitment then became apparent and could not have been solved without the invaluable and continuing assistance of the National Round Table Organization of Great Britain and Ireland. With their assistance about 150 volunteer donors have been HLA typed weekly by our laboratory since 1975 and now exceeds 50,000 names, our original target. Briefly, each Table recruits in its own area for periods ranging from weeks to a few months, having arranged the recruiting publicity, evening clinics for taking blood samples and bringing the samples to the HLA laboratory on the next morning. At present, the ultimate object is to reach 60,000 names, essentially to allow for wastage due to change of address, illness, retirements etc. Unfortunately, despite the increasing number of successful unrelated BMTps – financial support of the register still depends almost entirely on public donations. This effectively limits further expansion and long term research.

All the donors have been typed for the commoner HLA-A, -B and -C locus antigens from the initial blood sample. DR and A and B splits are identified if and when the HLA identical donor is recalled for a specific patient. A negative mixed lymphocyte reaction between donor and patient is usually taken to indicate optimal compatibility and is a prerequisite for eventual BMTp.

An initial report on the register in 1981 suggested that compatible unrelated siblings could be found for 29% of patients for whom a donor search had been made and that MLR negative donors were found for 75% of those patients with 10 or more potential donors (1). It was emphasized that the series investigated was too small for statistical evaluation.

Location of compatible donors

Initial requests for a donor search are received either from the patients' doctor (as in the UK) or from the patient's relatives (especially if from the USA). The HLA types of the patient are presented to the computer which identifies all donors with matching HLA types with and without compatible ABO identity. DR typing is undertaken at this stage to locate those identical and these are selected for MLR. Those donors with AB(C), DR and MLR identity are considered for BMTp. They are given a further option to withdraw at this stage from donating BM mainly in view of the small, but defined risk of the general anesthetic.

Functions of the panel

These may be summarized as follows:

a) To provide healthy unrelated donors for BMTp matching on HLA-A, -B (-C), -DR loci and with a negative reaction on MLC.
b) To provide support for BMTp patients with HLA matched platelets, granulocytes or ABO compatible blood. This is most appreciated during weekends or holiday periods when blood transfusion services are less easily available.
c) To provide amenable donors for research projects in which HLA and associated data is particularly relevant e.g. disease association studies etc.

In the main, the intention is to use the register to assist any patient who needs a BMTp regardless of geographical location, colour or creed. However, the expenses incurred have to be recovered from the requesting centre, doctor or patient, and provided these and all legal formalities can be agreed, the donors in general are prepared to travel abroad when necessary.

RESULTS

Number of donors on register

Table I. Number of donors on register.

Year	Number of donors	Cumulative total
1974*	1540	1540
1975	5094	6634
1976	6041	12675
1977	4842	17517
1978	5419	22936
1979	6385	29321
1980	6722	36043
1981	6396	42439
1982	6219	48658
1983**	4875	53572

* From 1/8/1974.
** Projected.

Sex and age of donors: percentage of blood donors

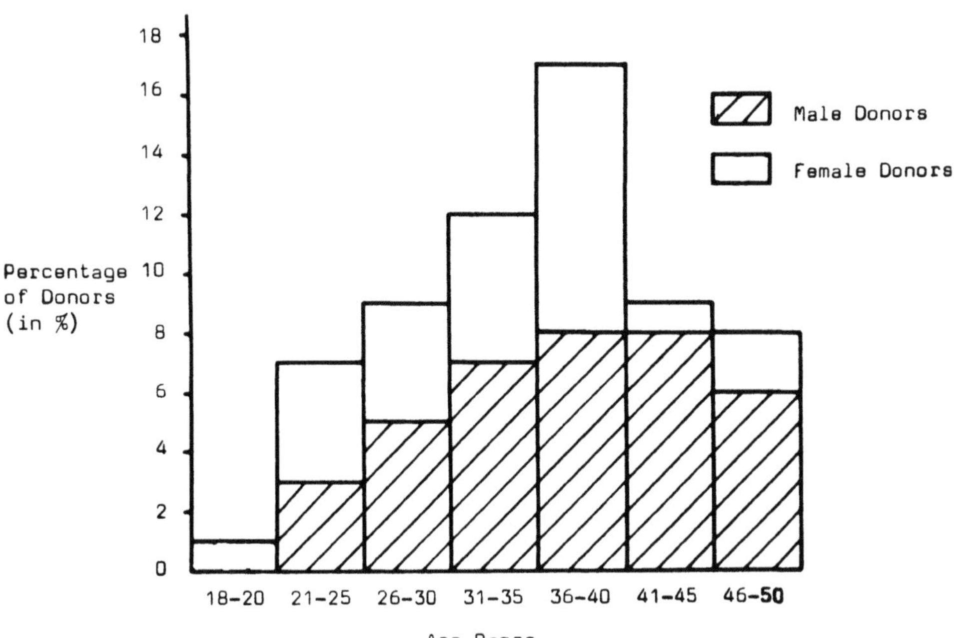

Figure 1. Age distribution of male/female donors on register.

Figure 1 shows that between the age limits for donor rècruitment (18–50 years) the highest donor response came from females aged 36–40 years; the highest male donor response occurred between 36 and 45 years old.

Table II.

Percentage of male/female donors on register:	
Percentage of female donors	63%
Percentage of male donors	37%
Percentage of blood donors/non blood donors on register:	
Percentage of blood donors	40%
Percentage of non blood donors	60%

The above data was calculated from a random sample of 400 donors on register.

In a random sample of 400 donors, 63% were females and of the total group 40% were registered blood donors.

Unrelated donor searches

a) Growth and distribution of requests for a donor search

Table III. Total, UK and overseas searches (1977 to 1983).

Year	Number of searches	UK searches	Overseas searches
1977	54	35	19
1978/9	105	81	24
1980	98	73	25
1981	108	61	47
1982	126	97	29
1983*	188	124	64

* Projected.

The number of searches as shown on Table III reflects the increasing interest in the possibility of using unrelated transplants and perhaps also increasing awareness of the existence of the panel.

Table IV shows that most non-British request came from the USA, but most countries with bone marrow transplant facilities are represented. No requests have yet come from Japan or the Eastern bloc except recently from Hungary.

b) Search of donor data

Of the 520 searches carried out between 1980 to 1983, 39,705 HLA identical donors were located by the computer. This makes an average of 130 searches per annum with a mean number of donors located of 9,926. However, in prac-

Table IV. Range of countries for which overseas searches were performed (1980 to 1983).

Country	Number of searches 1980*	1981	1982	1983**	Total searches	Percentage
USA	3	28	13	22	66	46
Australia	3	3	5	8	19	13
Canada	3	4	3	2	12	8.5
Italy	5	3	3	0	11	7.5
West Germany	1	6	0	2	9	6
France	1	0	3	4	8	5.5
Belgium	0	0	0	6	6	4.5
Switzerland	1	0	0	2	3	2
Finland	0	2	0	0	2	1.5
South Africa	0	0	2	0	2	1.5
India	0	0	0	2	2	1.5
Greece	0	0	0	2	2	1.5
The Netherlands	0	1	0	0	1	0.5
Denmark	0	0	0	1	1	0.5

* From 22/4/1980.
** To 14/10/1982.

Table V. Number of donors/search (1980 to 1983).

Total number of searches		520
Total number of donors		39705
Per annum:	Mean number of searches	130
	Mean number of donors	9926
Mean number of donors/search		76
Mean range of donors/search		0-679

tice more than 180 searches were carried out in 1983 which again reflects the trend. Finally, 76 donors were located per search with a range of 0–679 donors.

Table VI. Distribution of donors/search (1980 to 1983).

Range of donors/search	Percentage of searches
0	15
1-10	31
11-20	8.5
21-30	8
31-40	4.5
41-50	6
51-100	10
100+	17

Table VI shows the range of donors per search. Thus, 15% of searches produced no donors but 31% of patients had at least one donor (range 1–10). 33% had at least 41 donors (range 41–100+).

c) Donor/DR identity

During 1982 and 1983 (Nov) a total of 57 searches in which HLA identical donors had been found were followed up by DR typing of some of the donors.

Table VII. Percentage of donors DR typed who were DR identical with patient (1982/83).

	Number	Percentage
Donors DR typed	697	100
DR identical donors	68	9.76
DR non identical donors	629	90.24

Of 697 donors DR typed, 68 donors (9.76%) were DR identical with the patient. Thus an average of 10 HLA identical donors was found to provide 1 DR identical donor.

d) HLA/DR identity - relationship to MLR

Table VIII. Percentage of DR identical donors who were MLR negative (1982/83).

	Number	Percentage
DR identical donors MLR'd	39	100
MLR negative donors	9	23
MLR positive donors	30	77

In 18 donor searches reviewed, 39 HLA-A, -B and -DR identical donors were tested by MLR against the respective patient. 9 (23%) gave a negative reaction.

e) HLA/DR identical MLR negative donor frequency

Table IX. Theoretical number of donors/search required to find at least one matched donor for transplant.

Percentage of donors DR typed who are DR identical with patient = 9.76% Thus: 10.25 HLA identical donors required for 1 DR identical donor
Percentage of DR identical donors who are MLR negative = 23% Thus: 4.35 DR identical donors required for 1 MLR negative donor
Conclusion
Patients with 45+ donors/search will theoretically have at least one HLA/DR identical and MLR negative donor for transplant

Table IX summarizes the observed data in the series reviewed to find a fully compatible donor. Since 9.76% of HLA identical donors were found to be DR identical, then 10.25 HLA donors will be required to provide 1 DR identical donor.

Also, since 23% of DR identical donors were also MLR negative, then 4.35 DR identical donors are required to provide 1 MLR negative donor.

CONCLUSION

It can be concluded conservatively, that patients with 45 or more HLA identical donors will have at least one DR identical MLR negative donor for BMTp.

f) <u>The chances of finding a compatible BM donor from the register</u>

Table X. Percentage of patients for whom at least one matched donor can theoretically be found from register.

From 1982/83 searches	Percentage of searches with 0-44 donors	= 70%
	Percentage of searches with 45+ donors	= 30%

<u>Conclusion</u>

30% of patients will theoretically have at least one HLA/DR identical and MLR negative donor for transplant

Table X summarizes the review of searches carried out in 1982 and 1983.

30% of the patients had over 45 HLA identical potential donors. These patients should have at least one HLA/DR identical MLR negative donor for BMTp.

g) <u>Ratio of searches with < and > 45 donors/patient</u>

Table XI.

Year	% searches with 0–44 donors	% searches with 45+ donors
1980	68	32
1981	75	25
1982	70	30
1983	66	34
	279	121
Overall mean	70	30

Table XI shows that 30% of searches have 45 or more donors.
Thus: 30% of patients will theoretically have at least one HLA/DR identical and MLR negative donor.

DISCUSSION

The results obtained so far support our previous report which concluded that 29% of the patients initially referred for BMTp could be offered compatible unrelated donors (1). The report reviewed a series of 52 patients for whom 18 donors (29%) who were HLA-A and -B identical, MLR negative had been located. The MLR results suggested that where a patient had over 10 HLA identical donors then a donor showing negative mixed lymphocyte reactivity could be expected in 75% of cases.

The present larger series of searches suggests that this view may be over optimistic since it was found that complete compatibility i.e. HLA-A, -B, DR identity with MLR negativity could not be expected unless the patient had about 45 HLA identical donors. Nevertheless, 30% of the present series of 520 patients did have over 45 such donors on the register and thus the end result agrees with the previous report – namely that about 30% of patients can expect to have a donor almost with certainty. In the original report batches of donor sera were tested by MLR to establish compatibility with the patient – facilities for DR typing not being available (1). The assumption that DR identity between patient and donor could eliminate the need for the MLR test is clearly not justified; 75% of donors with identical DR antigens were found to give an unacceptably high MLR result against the patient. However, preliminary DR typing reduces the demands on the MLR laboratory since DR non-identity predictably results in a positive MLR result which can be avoided by this test. The significance of MLR-non reactivity still remains to be evaluated especially since it does not guarantee freedom from graft-versus-host disease (GvHD) even with compatible siblings.

However, despite the increasing interest in unrelated BMTps, too few have been carried out so far to evaluate their clinical importance: 3 patients (one with acute myeloid leukemia and two with aplastic anemia) grafted some 3 years ago are alive and well. A further 2 patients (one with aplastic anemia in London and one with acute lymphoblastic leukemia in the USA) grafted in mid 1983 are still alive and well. All the donors were found from the register. The clinical hazards particularly of GvHD do not seem to be increased. Recovery of T-cell function may be somewhat slower than when a related donor graft has been used, but the evidence is as yet insufficient for evaluation.

The "success" (or otherwise) of the Anthony Nolan Register is frequently bracketed with the clinical results following BMTp using an unrelated donor and this to some extent is understandable. However in a practical sense, the success of the register is more correctly a matter of the speed and efficiency with which it can provide one or more fully compatible donors for a specific patient after a request has been made. The register and its operators have no control over the clinical outcome, which is more a combination of the expertise of the hematologist or oncologist and supportive colleagues, as well as a high standard of nursing care. Too often, and despite the statistical evidence already available, bone marrow transplantation is recommended at too late a stage – particularly in the case of unrelated grafts. Often it is a relative who pressurises the clinician to take some action rather than allow the patient to die because a matching sibling is not available. Only one in four of patients generally will find a family donor – the remainder must look elsewhere. The results using half-matched relatives do not seem to offer an acceptable alternative, except possibly in young patients with inborn errors of metabolism. There may well be some increase of administrative, legal and financial problems in finding unrelated donors but the unfortunate patients without a compatible sibling must be given a chance to survive no less advantageous than their more fortunate fellowmen and women. It is essentially for this group of patients that the present register was intended.

SUMMARY

1. A British register of 50,000 unrelated volunteer bone marrow donors is now in active operation.
2. It is available worldwide for all patients needing a bone marrow transplant (subject to compliance with the necessary legal and financial requirements).
3. A recent review shows that it can provide a compatible HLA-A, -B, -DR, MLC negative donor for over 30% of patients.
4. On average only one in four of HLA-A, -B, and -DR identical donors were found to give a negative reaction in mixed lymphocyte culture.
5. Three UK patients with unrelated grafts from the donor register are well 3 years later and a further two patients grafted in mid 1983 are also alive and well.

ACKNOWLEDGEMENTS

I am grateful to Mr Jeremy Evans BSc for collating the data, to Mrs E.M. Long for typing the manuscript and to the Anthony Nolan Appeal Trustees, supporters and staff without whom the register could not be maintained.

REFERENCE

1. James DCO. The Anthony Nolan unrelated bone marrow register. Proc 5th Europ Symp on Bone Marrow Transplantation in Europe (II) Edited by Touraine J-L, Gluckman E, Griscelli C. Amsterdam-Oxford-Princetown: Excerpta Medica, 1981.

DEVELOPMENTS AND LIMITATIONS IN LIVER PRESERVATION

K. Rolles, R.Y. Calne

INTRODUCTION

Ten years ago progress in the field of organ transplantation could be predicted to come from four principle fields of research: tissue typing, donor specific immunosuppression, non-specific immunosuppression and organ preservation.

Tissue typing in the eyes of most clinical transplant surgeons has not lived up to its original promise. Donor specific immunosuppression is still only feasible in certain strains of rodents. The recent advances have perhaps predictably come from the field of non-specific immunosuppression. As far as organ preservation is concerned, nothing of clinical importance has emerged from this quarter in the last ten years.

Preservation of organs for clinical transplantation remains severely limited and techniques are quite empirical. Deprived of its blood supply an organ or tissue will suffer ischemic damage. The brain will suffer permanent loss of function after just a few minutes ischemia, whereas the skin can maintain its integrity and function after several hours' ischemia. Traditionally, it has been thought that the liver parenchyma is highly sensitive to damage from normothermic ischemia and is probably next in order of vulnerability to the central nervous system. The view has been that total interruption of the liver's blood supply at 37°C for more than 15 minutes will lead to impaired function and that the damage will become serious if the ischemic interval is prolonged beyond 30 minutes. This view has recently been challenged by the experiments of Feindal et al. (1). Pig livers were exposed to 60 minutes of normothermic ischemia by temporary hepatic artery clamping and insertion of a portojugular shunt. These manoeuvres reduced hepatic blood flow by 90% as judged by 127-Xenon washout studies. They reported only minimal transient changes in liver function tests following this procedure. Further experiments by Harris et al. (2) using the same model and technique showed that the period of warm ischemia could be extended to 90 minutes with uniform survival, but at 180 minutes, some deaths were recorded from liver failure. These authors pointed out that the traditional view of the liver being very sensitive to warm ischemia was based on work in the dog by Raffuci and Wangensteen (3), Hines and Roncoroni (4) and Farkouh et al. (5). Part of the explanation for this remarkable species difference may be that ischemia to the dog liver results in contraction of hepatic vein sphincters leading to hepatic venous obstruction and intense congestion of the liver on revascularisation, a phenomenon not seen in the pig or man.

However, whatever the warm ischemic tolerance of the livers of various species is, hepatic allografting, both experimental and clinical, should be performed only under optimal conditions with minimal warm ischemia.

EXPERIMENTAL PRESERVATION

Preservation of the liver poses problems far more formidable than with the kidney. Similar to the heart graft, the liver must function immediately on implantation as no effective form of artificial liver support exists. The literature of experimental liver preservation is extensive, but the relevance of much of this work to clinical practice is small. There is only one test of liver preservation acceptable to clinicians, and that is the immediate life sustaining function of the transplanted organ. It should be stressed that maintenance of elaborate cellular and excretory functions of the excised liver often for many hours, have not usually correlated with the ability of the preserved organ to support life.

Hypothermia remains the basic and most important factor in the preservation of solid organs. Cooling of an organ will reduce oxygen consumption and other metabolic functions in an exponential fashion. For every 10°C fall in temperature, oxidative metabolism is approximately halved. Levy (6) showed that at 5°C oxygen consumption in the dog kidney is less than 5% of normal. Schloerb et al. (7) found that for effective preservation cooling requires to be in the range 0°C–10°C, while cooling to temperatures above 25°C was ineffective (8).

Using surface and intraportal cooling with heparinized Ringer's solution at 4°C, both Starzl (9,10) and Moore (11) showed that life sustaining dog liver allografts would result only if the period of cold ischemia was less than 2 hours. A similar technique using Hartmann's solution for rapid cooling and a plasma based solution to stay "in situ" during the preservation period allowed Calne et al. (12) to preserve pig livers for 5–8 hours. Successful experimental preservation at 24 hours was reported by Lambotte et al. (13) using Isoproterenol to pretreat the donor and recipient and Collin's solution for preservation of the liver. The longest successful experimental liver preservation has been reported by Monden and Fortner (14) in the dog. Using flush cooling with Ringer's lactate followed by Sack's II solution containing prostacyclin, they have obtained life supporting function after 48 hours' storage.

Hypothermic perfusion techniques have been used by a number of workers, but the results do not appear to be superior to those of flush cooling. Brettschneider et al. (15) added hyperbaric oxygen to hypothermic perfusion with diluted blood and obtained successful preservation at 24 hours. Kamada (16) has recently reported similar times in the rat using a perfusion system employing a fluorocarbon emulsion as perfusate.

In an attempt to simplify the complicated and bulky apparatus necessary for continuous hypothermic perfusion with or without hyperbaria, Schalm et al. (17) and later Calne et al. (18) investigated low pressure trickle perfusion using a plasma protein perfusate and achieved successful preservation up to 11 hours. This period was extended to 17 hours by using an intermittent "squirt" perfusion technique using a similar perfusate with an acid pH.

On considering the varied experimental approaches and their respective safe preservation periods, we have taken the view that for our clinical programme, the simpler the preservation technique, the better.

CLINICAL EXPERIENCE

Over the 15 years of our programme 141 orthotopic liver allografts have been performed. Because of the restrictions implicit in liver preservation, we and all other units have employed two teams of surgeons, one for the donor procedure and one for the recipient operation, who usually work simultaneously, thus minimizing the preservation time of the graft.

In donor assessment and selection, we feel that all liver donors should be ventilated cases with an intact circulation in whom irreversible cerebral injury has led to a diagnosis of brain death. There is no longer a place for the use of non-heart beating cadavers in liver transplantation. Ventilation and circulation at near normal blood pressure should be maintained throughout the donor dissection if organs of optimal quality are to be obtained.

When the donor dissection is complete, liver cooling in situ is commenced via the portal vein with one litre of Hartmann's solution, containing 1000 units of Heparin at 4°C. To follow this 400–600 ml of plasma protein fraction also at 4°C, and containing certain additives is instilled before the liver is finally excised, and placed in a bowl of ice cold normal saline. The bowl and liver are then packed away in ice for storage and transportation.

This technique has enabled us to preserve human livers for up to 10.5 hours followed by immediate life sustaining function. However, if the donor has been hypotensive or if there have been technical difficulties in organ removal, then 10 hours of cold ischemia may be too long for safe transplantation, and 6 hours or less would be more realistic. Nevertheless, the preservation techniques used by Starzl – Collin's solution, and the Groningen group of Krom – Eurocollins, and our own method all allow approximately six to eight hours safe preservation and a travelling time of about 3 hours from the donor hospital to the transplant centre.

One important complication too frequently seen in the past in the King's College Hospital at Cambridge series but rarely encountered in Starzl's series was the problem of biliary sludge, in the absence of any mechanical obstruction to bile drainage. Biliary sludge presents as recurrent episodes of cholangitis and obstructive jaundice. McMaster (19,20) showed that this sludge, similar in consistency to the meconium in meconium ileus, was composed almost entirely of collagen derived from necrotic biliary epithelium. He demonstrated that biliary epithelium became vulnerable to damage from some of the constituents of the bile, probably bile salts, when the liver was in hypothermic storage. Careful washing out of the biliary tract and gall bladder to remove as much bile as possible before the period of cold storage, was effective in preventing this preservation related injury. Since adopting this manoeuvre clinically, our incidence of early biliary sludge has become very small. It is interesting that Starzl has always opened the gallbladder and irrigated it to prevent mucosal necrosis (21).

In conclusion, it must be said that with the logistics of transporting livers for transplantation within the United Kingdom and Western Europe, we feel that the currently used preservation techniques are adequate and there is little motivation to achieve longer periods of storage, especially if these involve expensive complicated apparatus requiring much technical expertise for maintenance and operation.

REFERENCES

1. Feindal CM, Harper R, Wallace AC, Wall WJ. Tolerance of the liver to ischemia: an experimental study. Can J Surg 1981;24:147–9.
2. Harris KA, Wallace AC, Wall WJ. Tolerance of the liver to ischemia in pig. J Surg Res 1982;33:524–30.
3. Raffucci FL, Wangenstein DH. Tolerance of dogs to occlusion of entire afferent vascular inflow to the liver. In: Surgical Forum 1950. American College of Surgeons, 191. W.B. Saunders, Philadelphia and London, 1951.
4. Hines IR, Roncoroni M. Acute hepatic ischemia in dogs. Surg Gynae & Obs 1956;102:689–94.
5. Farkough EF, Daniel AM, Beaudoin JG, MacLean LD. Predictive value of liver biochemistry in acute hepatic ischemia. Surg Gynae & Obs 1971; 132:832–9.
6. Levy A. Oxygen consumption and blood flow in the hypothermic perfused kidney. Am J Physiol 1959;197:111–5.
7. Schloerb PR, Waldorf RD, Welsh JS. The protective effect of kidney hypothermia on total renal ischemia. Surg Gynae & Obs 1959;109:561–6.
8. Moyer JH, Heider C, Morris GC, Handley C. Hypothermia III. The effect of hypothermia on renal damage resulting from ischemia. Ann Surg 1957; 146:152–66.
9. Starzl TE, Kaupp HA, Brock DR, Lazarus RV, Johnson RE. Reconstructive problems in canine liver homotransplantation with special reference to the postoperative role of hepatic venous flow. Surg Gynae & Obs 1960; 111:733–43.
10. Starzl TE, Putnam CW. In: Starzl TE, ed. Experience in hepatic transplantation. London, Philadelphia and Toronto: WB Saunders, 1969:41–64.
11. Moore FD, Wheeler AB, Demissianos HV, et al. Experimental whole-organ transplantation of the liver and of the spleen. Ann Surg 1960;152:374–87.
12. Calne RY, Dunn DC, Gajo-Reyero R, Jadjiyannakis EJ, Robson AJ. Trickle perfusion for organ preservation. Nature (London) 1972;235:171–3.
13. Lambotte L, Pontegnie-Istace S, Otte JB, Kestens CJ. The effect of Isoproterenol and Collins' solution on the preservation of canine livers with simple cooling. Transplant Proc 1974;6:301–3.
14. Monden M, Fortner JG. Twenty-four- and 48-hour canine liver transplantation by simple hypothermia with prostacyclin. Ann Surg 1982;196:38–42.
15. Brettschneider L, Daloze PM, Huguet C, et al. The use of combined preservation techniques for extended storage of orthotopic liver homografts. Surg Gynae & Obs 1968;126:263–75.
16. Kamada N, Calne RY, Wight DGD, Lines JG. Orthotopic rat liver transplantation after long-term preservation by continuous perfusion with fluorocarbon emulsion. Transplantation 1980;30:43–8.
17. Schalm SW, Terpstra JL, Drayer B, Van den Berg L, Veltkamp JJ. Simple method for shorter preservation of a liver homograft. Transplantation 1969;8:877–81.
18. Calne RY, Dunn DC, Herbertson BM, et al. Liver preservation by single passage hypothermic "Squirt" perfusion. Br Med J 1972;4:142–4.
19. McMaster P, Herbertson BM, Cusick C, Calne RY, Williams R. Biliary sludging following liver transplantation in man. Transplantation 1978; 25:56–62.
20. McMaster P. Bile studies after liver transplantation. Ann Roy Coll Surg of Eng 1979;61:435–40.
21. Starzl TE, Putnam CW. Donor hepatectomy and liver preservation. In: Starzl TE, ed. Experience in hepatic transplantation. London, Philadelphia and Toronto: WB Saunders, 1969:43–4.

NEW DEVELOPMENTS IN KIDNEY PRESERVATION

G. Kootstra, B.G. Rijkmans, W.A. Buurman, Th.J.M. Ruers, J.P. van Hooff

INTRODUCTION

When one overlooks the history of kidney preservation, it is impressive what has been reached in a period of just thirty years, assuming that the real kidney preservation started with the introduction of hypothermia. In 1952 Lefebre and Nizet (1) introduced cold storage aiming at a reduction of cellular metabolism. They cooled the kidney by immersing it in a cold solution (surface cooling). Flushing of the vascular tree of the kidney with a cold solution was introduced by Pegg and Calne (2) in 1963 and a preservation period of 24 hours in the dog model was reached. In the USA Humphries (3) worked on machine preservation and reached 48 hours in 1964. In 1967 Belzer (4) introduced cryoprecipitated plasma as perfusate in a modified machine constructed by him and his co-workers. Since their work cadaveric kidney transplantation is performed on an elective basis. Two years later, Collins (5) introduced the hyperosmolar solution for simple cold storage and it is this method, slightly modified as Eurocollins, that has reached overwhelming popularity in Europe. In the USA machine preservation has been the method of choice since Belzer's publication, though since the retrospective study of Opelz and Terasaki (6), published in 1978, stating that no advantage of machine preservation over cold storage could be established, the scene in the USA is changing towards cold storage. At the end of this bird's-eye survey of the development of preservation – far too short and not given credit to all the work performed – the question can be posed: How good then is this cold storage?

COLD STORAGE

The principle of the hyperosmolar and hyperkalemic flush and preservation solution is the prevention of cell swelling caused by ion shifts across the cell membranes. The kidney is stored at 0–4°C, assuming that metabolism at this temperature is so low that irreversible damage does not occur. It relies on physical means to prevent the harmful effects of ischemia and cooling. There is though some metabolism at this temperature and therefore limit in maximum preservation time. Initially 36 hours of cold preservation time was considered to be safe in the clinical situation. Several reports (7,8) have shown that preservation times of over 40 hours can be realized. In our transplant programme the mean cold storage time is 35.4 hours, and one out of three cadaveric kidneys transplanted has a cold storage time of 40 hours or more, with an overall immediate function rate of 70%. Indeed, cold storage is safe, simple, cost effective and suitable for transport.

It offers the opportunity to improve kidney transplant programmes from emergency day and night work into elective, well planned and prepared procedures. So, why to invest more energy into preservation research?

NEED FOR FURTHER RESEARCH IN THE FIELD OF PRESERVATION

One of the shortcomings of Eurocollins is, that it does not reduce the incidence of delayed function. The rate of delayed function has been reported to be as high as 50%. However, the cause of delayed function does not depend on the preservation technique alone; it is multifactorially determined (Table I).

Table I. Factors contributing to post-transplant function of kidneys.

	Factor
Donor age	a
Circulatory state of the donor	b
Surgical technique of donornephrectomy	c
Preservation method	d
Circulatory state of the recipient	e
Surgical technique of implantation	f
Immunological state of the recipient	g
Sum = a + b + c + d + e + f + g	

Sum of all factors determines post-transplant function.

In the management of transplant patients treated with the new immunosuppressive drug Cyclosporin it is of importance that there is direct post-transplant function. This requires a preservation method that has a very low incidence of delayed, c.q. non function.

The ideal preservation method corrects negative influences of the donor situation: i.e. a kidney damaged by ischemia in the donor is preserved in such a way that the damage is reversed and the kidney improves during the preservation procedure. It is evident that such a preservation method needs active metabolism, which is not provided in the cold storage procedure. The clinical relevance of such a preservation method is evident. There is a persisting shortage of kidneys for transplantation. This makes it necesary to accept less than ideal kidneys for transplantation. Sufficient numbers of cadaveric kidneys can be reached by the use of non-heart beating donors, i.e. the harvesting of kidneys from persons brought in dead into emergency rooms. If in The Netherlands the kidneys of 5% of the accident-victims could be harvested, shortage would not exist any longer. However, in these donors warm ischemia (defined as the time between cardiac arrest and flushing of the kidneys with a cold solution) is considerable and with Eurocollins the immediate functioning rate would be low; this could be a contra-indication for the further introduction of Cyclosporin.

A new development is going on in the research laboratory of Belzer (9) in Madison, Wisconsin, USA. They use in machine preservation a new perfusate, that maintains high levels of cortex tissue ATP. The new materials in the standard Belzer perfusate are adenosine and KH_2PO_4. Maintenance of high levels of ATP has two purposes. It may be important to stabilize lysosomes, mitochondria and cellular membranes and it may protect the kidney by a mechanism related to both the energy metabolism and cell swelling. Belzer's new perfusate was introduced in the clinical situation in May, 1982. The team in Madison procures kidneys after cardiac arrest, and therefore in a series of 77 cadaveric kidneys the mean warm ischemia time was 24 minutes, with a range from 0–50 minutes. The average cold ischemia time was 34 hours and ranged from 22–58 hours.

Sixty-two of the 77 kidneys transplanted (80.5%) had immediate function and another eight required only one posttransplant dialyses for hyperkalemia. When legal obstacles could be removed, a clinical trial with kidneys harvested from accident victims preserved with this new perfusate would be a crucial step in the reduction of the shortage of kidneys.

Fisher et al. (10) introduced retrograde oxygen persufflation (ROP) as a supplement to cold storage. The persufflation with oxygen is performed via cannulation of the renal vein. Bubbles of gas are allowed to escape through multiple needle puncture perforations in the renal capsule. The benificial effect was confirmed by Ross and Escott (11) in Melbourne and is now in study in Cambridge, in experiment and clinic. In canine experiments 48 hours preservation of one hour warm ischemia kidneys was successful, while non-persufflated kidneys did not function sufficiently to support life (12).

So two new developments can be recognized, aiming to reduce the harmful effect of warm ischemia.

Our research has been directed toward prolongation of the time of preservation to allow either induction of specific tolerance or to improve and introduce new matching techniques in cadaveric transplantation. Sofar, cold storage preservation in experimental work over 72 hours has been unsuccessful, while with machine preservation 96 hours is the safe limit. All studies over four days have sofar been only partially successful, with success rates dropping to one surviving dog out of three at seven or eight days of preservation.

The longest preservation time so far has been reached by Cohen and Johnson (13), who preserved ten dog kidneys for eight days (Table II). Two out of the ten had life-sustaining function, the remaining eight died of uremia. Woods (14) succeeded in two experiments to preserve one kidney for seven days, Liu (15) had three successes out of five, Cohen (16) two out of five and Ozaki (17) had no life-sustaining kidney out of four cases. In total, there are reports on 16 kidneys, preserved for seven days. Only six were life-sustaining, i.e. an overall success rate of 38%.

Six days preservation experiments have been published by our group (18). After hypothermic perfusion only one out of six dogs survived with poor kidney function.

Five day preservation has been studied by Ozaki (17) where two out of nine dogs had life-sustaining function and Cohen and Johnson (16), who obtained in 13 out of 27 experiments life-sustaining function. Toledo-Rereyra (19) obtained two surviving dogs out of 16 and Woods (14) one out of two.

It seems that in a five day preservation model less than half of the experiments will result in successful preservation.

Four day preservation experiments have a higher success rate. We have published life-sustaining function in six out of six experiments in the four

Table II. Results of experimental hypothermic continuous perfusion reported by serveral authors.

Author	Number of days	Type of machine	Perfusate	Survivors out of total number
Cohen GL, Johnson RWG (13)	8	Modified Belzer	Plasma protein fraction phosphate buffer added frusemide premedication	2 out of 10
Woods JE (14)	7	Belzer type machine	Belzer plasma high dose steroids added	1 out of 10
Liu WP et al. (15)	7	Travenol/Viacell	Human plasma protein fraction	3 out of 5
Cohen GL et al. (16)	7	Modified Belzer	Plasma protein fraction	2 out of 5
Ozaki A (17)	7	Senko machine (non-pulsatile roller pump, membrane oxygenator)	Modified Belzer's plasma (amino acid solution instead of mannitol)	0 out 0f 4
Rijkmans BG et al. (control group) (18)	6	Gambro	Kabi albumin	1 out of 6
Cohen GL et al. (16)	5	Modified Belzer	Plasma protein fraction	13 out of 27
Ozaki A et al. (17)	5	see above	see above	2 out of 4
Toledo-Pereyra LH (19)	5	Mox 100	Fibrinogen free	0 out of 8
			Belzer's plasma (Silica gel fraction)	2 out of 8
Woods JE (14)	5	see above	see above	1 out of 2

day preservation setting (18,20). The before mentioned eight, seven, six, five and four day preservation studies were all realized with mechanical perfusion techniques. Nearly all groups used different machines and perfusates (Table II). It seems unlikely that changes either in the machine or in the perfusate will improve results: four day hypothermic perfusion can be performed with a close to 100% success rate, while results of longer preservation are less consistent. Successful preservation for seven or eight days appeared to be an exception; the results were unpredictable and irreproducible!

We studied the effect of a normothermic blood perfusion halfway the period of hypothermic preservation. We assume that after four days hypothermic preservation, a kidney is "exhausted" which will lead to irreversible damage.

Just before complete exhaustion the kidney is recharged like a battery on the main by a normothermic blood perfusion. The supposition is that a recharged kidney can sustain another period of cold ischemia.

PREVIOUS WORK ON THE MODEL

In the first study we developed an ex-vivo perfusion system. Halfway the preservation period the kidney was perfused extracorporeally on the donor dog during four hours. This was effective in reducing the mean serum creatinine peak after four days kidney preservation (21). Then we proved the ex-vivo perfusion to work in a six day setting: in the control group without ex-vivo perfusion there was one survivor out of six dogs, while in the ex-vivo perfused group five out of six dogs had life-sustaining function (18,20).

The ideal time for the ex-vivo perfusion was studied and it turned out that the beneficial effect was reached at a three hours perfusion time (22). In this group six out of six kidneys survived with good kidney function. The next important step was the construction of a heart-lung machine that could replace the donor dog in the ex-vivo perfusion. A roller pump with bubble oxygenator was unsuccessful in providing the beneficial effect (unpublished data), a cylinder film oxygenator and a Dale Shuster-type pump resulted in three out of eight life-sustaining kidneys (23). This result was considered insufficient and a new machine was constructed. It combined the Dale Schuster-type pump with a membrane oxygenator. Hypothermic perfusion in combination with normothermic perfusion in this machine was studied in a controlled experiment:

Control group. In the control group of eight dogs with hypothermic perfusion only the kidneys were preserved for six days by hypothermic perfusion in a Gambro machine (Lund, Sweden) using a Kabi albumin perfusate at 5–7°C. The composition of the perfusate has been reported previously (21). After one hour hypothermic perfusion the perfusate pressure was adjusted to 20 mm Hg.

Experimental group. In the experimental group of 11 dogs the hypothermic perfusion of the kidneys was identical as in the control group. However, on the third day of the preservation period the kidneys were perfused in the heart-lung machine at 38°C. The heart-lung machine was primed with fresh alloblood (10 ml/g kidney weight). The blood donor dog was anesthetized with nembutal, and treated with 400 IU heparine/kg body weight and 1 g amoxicilline. The carotic artery of the donor dog was cannulated and the venous reservoir of the heart-lung circuit was filled rapidly. The perfusion of the preserved kidney started within two minutes after priming of the circuit. After three hours blood perfusion the kidneys were flushed with Eurocollins at 4°C and perfused in the Gambro machine with the same perfusate for the rest of the six day perservation period.

In the control and in the experimental group the kidneys were tested for (life-sustaining) function by transplantation to the neck of the donor dog and immediate contralateral nephrectomy.

RESULTS

Survival and function after implantation. In the blood perfused group all kidneys regained normal colour upon revascularisation and produced urine immediately. Nine out of 11 dogs of the blood perfused group survived in healthy condition. Two dogs had to be sacrificed at respectively day three and seven after implantation because of wound dehiscence and urine leakage respectively. The serum creatinine of these two dogs followed the pattern of the others in the experimental group, compatible with functional recovery. In the blood perfused group the mean serum creatinine concentration returned to normal within two weeks after implantation and had a maximum value of 533 μmol/l on day two (range 279–885 μmol/l).

In the control group with only continuous hypothermic perfusion the kidneys also regained their normal colour upon revascularisation. However, the urine production was low. In the control group only one out of eight dogs survived; the others died uremic within five days. The only survivor reached a maximum serum creatinine concentration of 1080 μmol/l on day five. In contrast to data reported by other authors (16,17), the histological sections of both groups showed normal glomeruli and vessels. Signs of endothelial damage leading to intravascular coagulation and fibrin thrombi in the glomular capillaries have not been observed. This so called "perfusion nephropathy" following hypothermic continuous perfusion has been described by several authors (24,25). It has been suggested that perfusion nephropathy can be prevented by low perfusion pressure in hypothermic perfusion (26) as applied in our experiments. The kidneys of the control group showed severe tubular damage, many casts were observed. In the perfused group, however, relatively well preserved tubules were observed in the kidneys of the two cases with technical failure.

Although the exact mechanism of the beneficial effect of the blood perfusion on the kidneys remains sofar unknown, the histological data suggest a recovery of tubular cells during the blood perfusion at normothermia.

From this study it can be concluded that it is possible to prevent preservation damage by three hours normothermic isolated blood perfusion after which the organ can be preserved for another three days. Furthermore, by using an artificial perfusate it would be possible to find out which factors are responsible for the beneficial effect of the intermediate perfusion. This might also contribute to the development of improved hypothermic preservation techniques.

Finally, the good results of these six day preservation experiments suggest that the application of alternating hypothemic and normothermic perfusion might enable intermediate kidney preservation in the clinical situation.

REFERENCES

1. Lefebre L, Nizet E. Shunt vasculaire dans les reins de chiens perfusés et conservés a basse temperature. Arch Int Pharmacol 1952;92:119–27.
2. Pegg DE, Calne RY, Pryse-Davies J, Leigh-Brown F. Canine renal preservation using surface and perfusion cooling techniques. Ann NY Acad Sci 1964;120:506–23.
3. Humphries AL, Russel R, Gregory J, Carter RH, Moretz WH. Hypothermic perfusion of the canine kidney for 48 hours followed by reimplantation. Am Surg 1964;30:748–52.
4. Belzer FO, Ashby BS, Dunphy JE, 24-hour and 72-hour preservation of canine kidneys. Lancet 1969;ii:536–9.
5. Collins GM, Bravo-Shugarmon M, Terasaki PI. Kidney preservation for transplantation. Lancet 1969;ii:1219–22.
6. Opelz G, Terasaki PI. Advantage of cold storage over machine perfusion for transplantation of cadaver kidneys. Transplantation 1982;33:64–8.
7. Squifflet JP, Pirson Y, Gianello P, Van Caugh P, Alexandre GPJ. Safe preservation of human renal cadaver transplants by Eurocollins solution up to 50 hours. Transplant Proc 1981;XIII:693–6.
8. Abouna GM, Kumar AS, White AG, et al. Experience with imported human cadaveric kidneys having unusual problems and transplanted after 30–60 hours of preservation. Transplant Proc 1984;XVI:61–3.
9. Belzer FO. Transplant Proc 1984;XVI:161–3.
10. Fisher JH, Czerniak H, Hauer U, Isselhard W. A new simple method for optimal storage of ischemically damaged kidneys. Transplantation 1978; 25:362–4.
11. Ross H, Escott ML. Gaseous oxygen perfusion of the renal vessels as an adjunct in kidney preservation. Transplantation 1979;28:362–4.
12. Rolles K. Personal communication.
13. Cohen GL, Johnson RWG. Perfusate buffering for 8-day canine kidney storage. Proc Eur Soc Art Org 1980;VII:235–9.
14. Woods JE. Successful three-to-seven-day preservation of canine kidneys. Arch Surg 1971;102:614–7.
15. Liu WP, Humphries AL, Russell R, Stoddard LD, Garcia LA, Serkes KD. Three- and seven-day perfusion of dog kidneys with human plasma protein fraction IV-4. Surgical Forum 1973;24:316–8.
16. Cohen GL, Ballardie FW, Mainwaring A, Johnson RWG. Lysosomal enzyme release during successful 5-, 7- and 8-day canine kidney storage. In: Pegg DE, Jacobsen IA, Halasz NA, eds. Organ preservation: Basic and applied aspects. Lancaster-Boston-The Hague: MTP Press Ltd, 1982:249–53.
17. Ozaki A, Fukao K, Sano M, Okamura T, Iwasaki Y. Five-day preservation of canine kidneys using a preservation machine. In: Pegg DE, Jacobson IA, Halasz NA, eds. Organ preservation: Basic and applied aspects. Lancaster-Boston-The Hague: MTP Press Ltd, 1982:245–49.
18. Rijkmans BG, Van der Wijk J, Donker AJM, Slooff MJH, Kootstra G. Functional studies in 6 days successful preserved canine kidneys. J Urol 1982;127:163–5.

19. Toledo-Pereyra LH, Condie RM, Malmberg R, Simmons RL, Najarian JS. A fibrinogen-free plasma perfusate for preservation of kidneys for one hundred and twenty hours. Surg Gyn Obst 1974;138:901–6.
20. Van der Wijk J, Sloof MJH, Rijkmans BG, Kootstra G. Successful 96 and 144 hour experimental kidney preservation: A combination of standard machine preservation and newly developed normothermic ex-vivo perfusion. Cryobiology 1980;17:473–7.
21. Kootstra G, Van der Wijk J, Rijkmans BG. A new device towards intermediate term kidney preservation. An experimental study. Scand J Urol Nephrol (Suppl) 1980 ;54:86–9.
22. Van der Wijk J, Rijkmans BG, Kootstra G. Six day kidney preservation in a canine model. Influence of a 1 to 4 hr ex-vivo perfusion interval. Transplantation 1983;35:408–11.
23. Rijkmans BG, Kootstra G, Van der Wijk J, Nizet A. Intermediate ex vivo and in vitro perfusion to prolong hypothermic kidney preservation up to six days. In: Pegg DE, Jacobson IA, Halasz NA, eds. Organ preservation: Basic and applied aspects. Lancaster-Boston-The Hague: MTP Press Ltd, 1982:267–72.
24. Spector D, Limas C, Frost JL, et al. Perfusion nephropathy in human transplants. N Engl J Med 1976;295:1217–21.
25. Hill GS, Light JA, Perloff LJ. Perfusion-related injury in renal transplantation. Surgery 1976;79:440–7.
26. Cerra FB, Raza S, Andres GA, Siegel JH. The endothelial damage of pulsatile renal preservation and its relationship to perfusion pressure and colloid osmotic pressure. Surgery 1977;81:534–41.

PRESERVATION OF HEMOPOIETIC STEM CELLS

J.M. Goldman

INTRODUCTION

Hemopoiesis in mammals is maintained by continuing proliferation and differentiation of putative pluripotential hemopoietic stem cells (PHSC). Such cells cannot be recognized by morphological or immunological techniques but can be defined operationally in experimental systems and clinical studies. Their presence in normal bone marrow (and probably also in the peripheral blood), from which site they can be harvested by appropriate techniques, has formed the basis for treating patients with various types of hematological or neoplastic disease by transplantation of allogeneic or autologous bone marrow cells. In this paper I will attempt to define the PHSC, to describe some of the methods by which such cells may be collected for clinical use, to refer to methods for storing stem cells and outline the results of their use in clinical practice.

PLURIPOTENTIAL HEMOPOIETIC STEM CELLS

The modern era of experimental hematology began in 1961 with the demonstration by Till and McCulloch (1) that nucleated cells collected from the bone marrow of mice could on injection into heavily irradiated syngeneic animals restore hemopoiesis and prevent otherwise inevitable death. They showed moreover that the spleens of these "reconstituted" mice had nodules visible on their surface which on histological examination proved to be composed of myeloid cells. The cells that gave rise to these nodules or colonies were designated spleen colony-forming units (CFU-S) and were regarded for some years as equivalent to the PHSC responsible for reestablishing hemopoiesis in the murine marrow. Though a similar assay can be developed in rats, no equivalent splenic colonies are formed after marrow transplantation in other mammals or in man. It is now recognized that the CFU-S almost certainly has limited capacity for self-replication and may not therefore reflect the most immature or undifferentiated stem cell normally present in the mammalian marrow (2) (Fig. 1).

Attempts to develop an assay for human PHSC have hitherto been largely unsuccessful. In the early 1970s Pike and Robinson adapted the agar system for assaying granulocyte/macrophage committed colony-forming cells (3) and subsequently assays for erythroid- and megakaryocyte-committed progenitor cells have been developed. In 1978 Fauser and Messner reported modifications of a methyl cellulose assay system incorporating exogenous erythropoietin in which single colonies containing myeloid cells of more than one lineage could be identified (4). The originating cell was designated CFU-GEMM

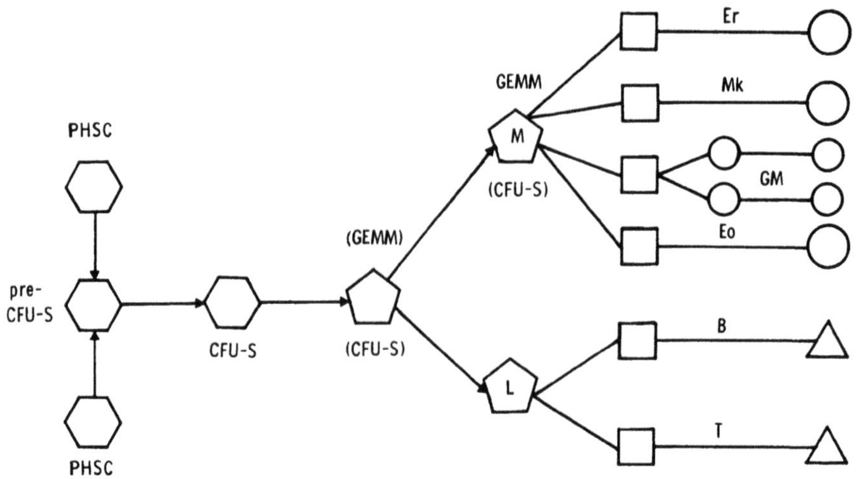

Figure 1. Schematic diagram showing relationship between pluripotential hemopoietic stem cells (PHSC) with the spleen colony forming cell (CFU-S) and the various myeloid (M) committed progenitor cells, GEMM (granulocyte/erythroid/macrophage/megakaryocyte), Er (erythroid), Mk (megakaryocytic), GM (granulocyte/macrophage) and Eo (eosinophilic). The Lymphoid (L) pathway is showing giving rise to cells of B and T lineages.

(granulocyte, erythrocyte, macrophage, megakaryocyte) and was regarded as representing a primitive myeloid progenitor or stem cell. However the capacity for continuing self-replication has not yet been convincingly demonstrated.

That stem cells with considerable self-replicative potential must be present in the marrow of normal man is amply documented by the success of allogeneic bone marrow transplantation. Thus a standard bone marrow harvest involves collection of between 1 and 2% of the total number of nucleated cells in an individual's marrow cavity. The transfer of these harvested cells to a suitable recipient can restore hemopoiesis which in some cases has lasted more than 10 years; although graft failure, thought in some cases to be immunologically determined, does occur, there is no suggestion that stem cell "exhaustion" is actually a major risk some years after grafting. Thus one may provisionally conclude that transfer of as little as 1% of a normal donor's stem cell stock can maintain hemopoiesis in the recipient perhaps indefinitely.

Human PHSC cannot be recognized by conventional morphological methods, partly because they are probably present in normal marrow in very low concentration and partly because they may closely resemble other cells, such as interphase or transitional lymphocytes. For the same reasons characterization of their cell surface characteristics, especially surface antigens, has not hitherto been possible. By extrapolation however from studies with experimental animals it is likely that human PHSC lack most of the conventional lymphoid and myeloid antigens and probably also lack HLA-DR surface determinants.

STEM CELL COLLECTION IN CLINICAL PRACTICE

In the late 1950s and through the 1960s a number of attempts were made to transplant marrow from normal donors to patients with leukemia, aplastic anemia or individuals accidentally exposed to high doses of ionizing radiation. These efforts were uniformly unsuccessful or inevaluable. There were at least three reasons for these early failures: the patients were for the most partly inadequately immunosuppressed, nothing was known of the importance of HLA matching and in most cases the numbers of nucleated cells transferred were relatively small.

In the late 1960s and early 1970s Thomas and his colleagues, first in Cooperstown New York and subsequently in Seattle, did much to establish the principles of successful allogeneic marrow in man (5). Thus it became clear that engraftment of marrow was most likely to occure and the risk of severe graft-versus-host disease (GvHD) was likely to be smallest if donor and recipient were HLA-identical sibs. It also appeared from analysis of data obtained mainly with transplantation for aplastic anemia that engraftment was most likely to occur if the transfusion contained at least 3.0×10^8 nucleated marrow cells per kilogram of the recipient's body weight, although smaller numbers e.g. 2.0×10^8, were still frequently effective. Because 10^5 normal marrow cells contain about 30 granulocyte/ macrophage committed progenitor cells (CFU-GM), one can calculate that 3.0×10^8 nucleated cells may include perhaps 9×10^4 CFU-GM but the equivalent numbers of PHSC is totally unknown.

For harvesting marrow the normal donor is usually given a general anesthetic but the procedure can be carried out conveniently with spinal anesthesia. Two operators using syringes and standard bone marrow aspirate or biopsy needles then collect from the donor's iliac bones about 1 litre of blood and suspended marrow cells. Routinely this material is anticoagulated with heparin and diluted with a tissue culture medium or other buffered physiological fluid before being filtered and transfused to the patient. Some groups have attempted to develop a totally "closed" system to maintain sterility but in practice an "open" system is far less cumbersome and the evidence that infection is introduced during the collection procedure is sparse. The procedure lasts typically between 45 and 90 minutes and leaves the donor with a sore back and mild anemia for some days but is usually otherwise uncomplicated. However in a small number of normal donors impressive complications, including local infections, cerebral infarction and cardiac arrest, have occurred and the procedure should not therefore be regarded as totally without risk. A death in a normal donor has recently been reported.

It is technically simpler and probably also safer to collect nucleated cells from the peripheral blood. CFU-S and CFU-GM are present in the blood of mice and CFU-GM circulate in man (6). Nucleated blood cells from a number of mammalian species can readily restore hemopoiesis in lethally irradiated syngeneic animals and by extrapolation one may presume that human blood also contains circulating PHSC, but in practice the evidence is none too persuasive. Thus an attempt to treat aplastic anemia with transfusions of nucleated blood cells from a normal identical twin failed when subsequent marrow transplantation was succesful (7) and attempts to expedite hematological recovery by autologous blood-derived stem cell transfusion after chemotherapy for Ewing's sarcoma were also unsuccessful (8). Patients or normal donors can nonetheless be subjected to leukapheresis with a continuous flow blood cell separator and large numbers of nucleated cells can be collected and cryopreserved (9,10). Whether such an approach will ever replace the use of harvested bone marrow is uncertain.

STEM CELLS FOR ALLOGENEIC MARROW TRANSPLANTATION

Patients with aplastic anemia, immune deficiency syndromes and certain types of leukemia can in some cases be effectively treated by transplantation of allogeneic bone marrow cells. Patients with immune deficiencies can sometimes be grafted without preceding immune suppression but patients with aplastic anemia are conventionally treated with high doses of cyclophosphamide before transplant. For patients with leukemia pre-transplant treatment has the dual objectives of suppressing the immune system and destroying residual leukemic clone-forming cells. Such treatment usually includes cyclophosphamide and whole body irradiation although te combination of busulphan with cyclophosphamide has recently proved equally valuable (11). By such treatment perhaps as many as 60% of patients transplanted for acute myeloid leukemia in first remission can be cured; the cure rate for patients transplanted with acute lymphoblastic leukemia in first remission or for patients in the chronic phase of chronic granulocytic leukemia may be even higher.

It is remarkable that PHSC transfused intravenously to recipients "home" to appropriate sites in the bone marrow and reconstitute hemopoiesis relatively rapidly. In some patients we have however noted transient periods of splenomegaly following marrow transplantation and it is possible, though unproved, that myeloid cell proliferation occurs initially in the spleen and that hemopoiesis in the marrow only becomes fully functional a few days later. Whatever the truth of this supposition, the bone marrow examined 7 to 8 days after transplant already shows regenerating hemopoiesis with discrete foci of erythroid, granulocytic and megakaryocytic activity. The blood granulocyte count begins to rise by about day +8 and may exceed $1.0x10^8/l$ by day +12 or +14. Platelet numbers begin to rise after about 12 days but may not reach normal values until three or more weeks post-transplant. The rate of rise of lymphoid cell numbers is variable and affected by the nature of post-graft immunosuppression and by such treatment as may be necessary for GvHD. Total lymphoid cell numbers may be normal within three months of transplant but typically the helper-to-suppressor ratio of T-lymphocytes may remain abnormally low for some condiserable time.

So far as can be judged the kinetics of myeloid stem cell engraftment in HLA-identical sib transplants and in non-genotypically matched transplants (e.g. haplo-identical or matched unrelated donor-recipients relationships) are similar or identical. In the latter situation engraftment may occur rapidly but may also be associated with relatively severe GvHD or with marrow transplant "mismatch syndrome" (12).

STEM CELL CRYOPRESERVATION

It was shown more than 20 years ago that cyropreserved bone marrow cells stored for months or years would reconstitute hemopoiesis in lethally irradiated syngeneic or histocompatible animals. Corresponding recoveries of

CFU-S, CFU-GM and CFU-GEMM after various periods of cryopreservation support the general conclusion that under optimal conditions stem cells and progenitor cells survive remarkably well for long periods. These conditions are now reasonably well defined. Dimethyl sulphoxide (DMSO) at a concentration of about 10% is a better cryoprotectant for marrow stem cells than glycerol. The optimal rate of freezing is about 1°C per minute and there is no definite evidence that measures designed to counteract the release of latent heat of fusion are truly necessary. Below -40°C the rate of subsequent freezing may be safely increased but the viability of stem cells is better maintained if they are then stored at -196°C in liquid nitrogen rather than in mechanical freezers at -79°C.

For reconstitution the frozen cells are best thawed rapidly in a 37°C waterbath; there is still some uncertainty as to whether DMSO must be diluted out slowly or whether indeed its removal is unnecessary before transfusion of cells to the patient. Whatever the answer the administration of relatively small amounts of DMSO intravenously is probably not harmful.

Where marrow has been collected as part of a programme of autografting in the management of a patient with acute leukemia or a solid tumor, cryopreservation will not be necessary if the schedule of chemotherapy or chemoradiotherapy can be completed within 48 or 72 hours. In this case bone marrow cells can be stored in a refrigerator at 4°C with every expectation that the PHSC will retain their viability.

MARROW-DERIVED STEM CELLS FOR AUTOGRAFTING

The use of autologous hemopoietic stem cells in the management of patients with neoplastic disease depends on the assumption that the administration of high doses of cytotoxic drugs or of cytotoxic drugs plus irradiation may eradicate the tumor but would be unduly hazardous if restoration of marrow function could not be expedited with the autograft (13). Thus there are two practical considerations: how best to treat the patient for maximal tumor cell kill and how to manipulate the marrow in vitro if there is a reasonable likelihood that harvested marrow cells are contaminated with tumor stem cells. It is worth noting that such marrow "purging" or "decontamination" would be totally unncessary a) if the harvested marrow did not in practice contain tumor stem cells, b) if tumor stem cells were selectively damaged by the cryopreservation procedure, or c) if small numbers of tumor stem cells reinoculated into the patient were inadequate to reestablish the tumor. Some of the possible approaches to marrow purging in vitro are listed in Table I. Ritz and his colleagues have recently reported details of the successful use of a monoclonal antibody with complement lysis to free harvested marrow of residual acute lymphoblastic leukemia cells (14); their experimental design does not allow the reader to draw firm conclusions about the clinical value of the purging procedure but the treated bone marrow was clearly able to restore hemopoiesis and a number of their patients have become 2-year disease-free survivors.

BLOOD-DERIVED STEM CELLS FOR AUTOGRAFTING

The number of circulating CFU-GM can be increased in the peripheral blood of man by various manipulations including exercise and the administration

Table 1. Possible methods for "purging" or "decontaminating" marrow that may contain residual neoplastic cells.

Physical methods	Cell size Cell density Heat sensitivity
Pharmacological methods	Deoxycoformycin 4-hydroperoxycyclophosphamide Asta Z 7557 Lysosomotropic detergents
Immunological methods	Conventional antibodies Monoclonal antibodies single, C^1-fixing in combination coupled with cytotoxic drugs coupled with toxins, e.g. ricin coupled with magnetized particles

including exercise and the administration of cytotoxic drugs and other pharmacological agents. This does not however necessarily imply that PHSC are also induced to enter the circulation in increased numbers and efforts to demonstrate such cells in the circulaton have been inconclusive (see above). The situation may however be very different in patients with chronic myeloid leukemia (CML). This disease may uniquely represent a situation in which PHSC are immortalized and thereby increased very greatly in number both in the marrow and in the peripheral blood. Studies in the 1970s have shown conclusively that PHSC collected from the peripheral blood of untreated patients are capable of restoring hemopoiesis in patients treated with "supralethal" chemoradiotherapy in the attempt to control the blastic phase of the disease (15,16). A recent analysis of results of this approach in the management of CML showed that the median duration of survival after chemotherapy and blood-derived stem cell autografting was 24 weeks with a range of 1 to 152 weeks (17). Thus the procedure can undoubtedly prolong life for some patients in transformation but cannot be regarded as a major advance in the management of this disease.

REFERENCES

1. Till JE, McCulloch EA. A direct measurement of the radiation sensitivity of normal mouse bone marrow cells. Radiat Res 1961;14:213–22.
2. Hodgson GS, Bradley TR. Properties of hemopoietic stem cells surviving 5-fluorouracil treatment: Evidence of a pre-CFUs cell? Nature 1979;281: 381–2.
3. Pike BL, Robinson WA. Human bone marrow colony growth in agar-gel. J Cell Comp Physiol 1970;76:77–84.
4. Fauser AA, Messner HA. Granuloerythropoeitic colonies in human bone marrow, peripheral blood and cord blood. Blood 1978;52:1243–7.
5. Thomas ED, Storb R, Clift RA, et al. Bone-marrow transplantation. New Engl J Med 1975;292:832–43 & 895–902.

6. McCarthy DM, Goldman JM. Transfusion of circulating stem cells. CRC Press 1984 (in press).
7. Hershko C, Gale RP, Ho WG, et al. Cure of aplastic anemia in paroxysmal nocturnal hemoglobinuria by marrow transfusion from identical twin: failure of peripheral-leukocyte transfusion to correct marrow aplasia. Lancet 1979;i:945–7.
8. Abrams RA, Glaubiger D, Appelbaum FR, et al. Result of attempted hemopoietic reconstitution using isologous, peripheral blood mononuclear cells: a case report. Blood 1980;56:516–20.
9. Richman CM, Weiner RS, Yankee RA. Increase in circulating stem cells following chemotherapy in man. Blood 1976;47:1031–9.
10. Lasky L, Ash RC, Kersey JH, et al. Collection of pluripotential hemopoietic stem cells by cytapheresis. Blood 1982;59:822–7.
11. Santos GW. 1983 Personal communication.
12. Powles RL, Morgenstern GR, Kay HEM, et al. Mistmatched family donors for bone marrow transplantation as treatment for acute leukemia. Lancet 1983;i:612–5.
13. Goldman JM, Nolasco I. The contribution of hemopoietic autografting in malignant disease. Exper Hemat (suppl 13) 1983;11:139–44.
14. Ritz J, Sallan SE, Bast RC, et al. Autologous bone marrow transplantation in CALLA-positive acute lymphoblastic leukemia after in vitro treatment with J5 monoclonal antibody and complement. Lancet 1982;ii: 60–3.
15. Goldman JM, Catovsky D, Hows J, et al. Cryopreserved peripheral blood cells functioning as autografts in patients with chronic granulocytic leukemia in transformation. Brit Med J 1979;1:1310–3.
16. Goldman JM, Catovsky D, Goolden AWG, et al. Buffy coat autografts for patients with chronic granulocytic leukemia in transformation. Blut 1981;42:149–55.
17. Haines A, Goldman JM, Worsley AM, et al. Chemotherapy and autografting for chronic granulocytic leukemia in transformation: Probable prolongation of survival for some patients. In preparation.

IS THE BASIS OF CLEANING AUTOLOGOUS BONE MARROW TRANSPLANTS IN LEUKEMIA STRONG ENOUGH?*

B. Löwenberg

INTRODUCTION

Bone marrow transplantation (BMT) from allogeneic donors following intensive chemotherapy and total body irradiation produces lasting remissions in a significant number of patients with acute lymphoblastic and myeloblastic leukemia (1–4). Autologous bone marrow transplantation (ABMT) in patients with acute leukemia may benefit from the same cytotoxic therapy. Its attractivity relates to the fact that each patient would have a donor, i.e. be his or her own donor, and that (in the absence of graft-versus-host disease) age restriction for transplantation is far less to be considered. On the other hand, ABMT is likely to involve a higher rate of leukemia relapse post transplantation. The first results of ABMT were obtained in end stage patients, and although they resulted in new remissions, these were usually of short duration (5). More recently several groups have started ABMT in patients with acute leukemia during their complete remission. This approach is foreseen to achieve a tumor cell killing due to: a) the pretransplant chemo- and radiotherapy; b) autologous bone marrow is probably contaminated with subclinical numbers of leukemic cells; the reinfusion of autologous bone marrow may result in a further decrease of tumor due to loss of cells in various tissues following intravenous administration (inappropriate seeding) (6–9); c) when purging methods are applied to the marrow graft, neoplastic cells may be successfully eliminated.

Information as regards the seeding and migration properties of AML cells following intravenous transfer has been gathered in animal models and its relevance to the human situation can only be verified in clinical trials. For this purpose, remission durations and survival after ABMT should be evaluated, relative to the results in allotransplant recipients.

CLINICAL RESULTS

Four patients with AML in first remission lacking a MHC compatible donor in the family, were grafted with cryopreserved bone marrow. This bone marrow had been collected autologously during remission. Before the infusion of the graft, they were treated with a high dose of cyclophosphamide (120 mg/kg body weight over 2 days) and total body irradiation (8 Gy; 7 Gy to the lungs). Serious post-transplant complications were not encountered. All were discharged from the hospital between day 30–70. One patient

* This work was supported by the Dutch Cancer Foundation "Koningin Wilhelmina Fonds".

had an AML relapse in the marrow and peripheral blood at 13 months post-transplantation and died one month later from progressive leukemia in spite of chemotherapy. The other three patients have been free of medical interventions and therapy and continue in first remission for a total of 4+ years, 2+ years and 7+ months. These experiences indicate that remission of encouraging durations may be obtained with autologous bone marrow grafts, which have not been freed of tumor cells.

PURGING OF AUTOLOGOUS MARROW TRANSPLANT AND TUMOR CELL HETEROGENEITY

Leukemia cells rarely share the same biophysical or immunological properties; they exhibit a phenotypic heterogeneity. The removal of tumor cells is therefore usually directed at subsets of the neoplasm and only contributes a therapeutic effect if the clonogenic cells are separated out.

In this respect the application of colony culture techniques may be useful. This may be of importance in order to define the cellular properties of these cells and monitor their presence or removal. AML colony forming cells during colony forming produce a progeny with meyloid markers on the surface, which suggests that AML cells may further mature in vitro (10). Also subsets with variable proliferative abilities can be distinguished, e.g. colony forming cells, macrocluster forming cells and microcluster forming cells which express a different degree of maturation (11). This had indicated that the heterogeneous cell composition of AML is a reflection of maturation within the tumor.

Additional in vitro studies indicate that AML clonogenic cells may exhibit specific phenotypes, different from those of other AML cells. The AML clonogenic cells were defined utilizing a number of monoclonal antibodies (against myeloid differentiation antigens) in complement mediated lysis and FACS cell sorting of colony forming cells. L-CFU express cell surface anti-

Table I. Phenotypic analysis of AML colony forming cells and "end cells" in colonies.

		Expression of marker	
McAb	(ref.)	L-CFU*	Colony and cells**
Ia	(10)	+	++/-
AT1	(10)	+	++/-
WT1	(12)	-	+/-
B4.3	(13)	-	+/-
S3-13	(14,15)	+	+
S4-7	(14,15)	+	+

* L-CFU were typed with a series of monoclonal antibodies before culture in complement lysis assays or FACS cell sorting.

** Colony cells were harvested at the time of maximal growth in the PHA-leukocyte feeder system (day 7), then resuspended and then studied in indirect immunofluorescence with the monoclonal antibodies.

Table II. Effect of colony method on L-CFU typing.

	Kill of L-CFU with McAb			
	Patient 1		Patient 2	
	anti Ia	B4.3	anti Ia	B4.3
PHA-1.f assay	+	+	-	-
Robinson assay	+	-	+	±

AML L-CFU were tested for expression of certain membrane markers in a complement lysis test using anti Ia and B4.3 McAb.
L-CFU surviving the cytotoxicity procedure were compared in two colony assays: the PHA leukocyte feeder method and the Robinson (double agar with leukocyte feeder) method.

gens at specific densities, which were different from those on other AML blast cells. These results are summarized in Table I. The data support the idea that a good understanding of the phenotypic variability of AML is essential for performing efficient purging of autologous marrow in transplantation. The approaches applied with monoclonal antibodies and without assaying for L-CFU may otherwise be laborious activities without a therapeutic effect. In a comparative analysis it also appeared (Table II) that a different colony assay may induce colony formation from different precursor cells and thus be selective. This means that the choice of the particular colony assay may be an important variable in monitoring tumor cell separation from marrow autografts. How these various colony forming cell populations relate to in vivo proliferative capacities has yet to be resolved.

CONCLUSION

Transplantation of non purified autologous marrow may give prolonged remissions in a significant number of patients with AML, when applied during first remission. It is of importance to note that the patients did not receive post-graft maintenance chemotherapy. Since the marrow graft is likely to be admixed with small numbers of tumor cells, it is supposed that ineffective seeding in various organs following infusion contributes to leukemia cell loss. The question whether tumor cell purging is necessary in all patients remains to be answered. Colony assays and a series of selected monoclonal antibodies were applied to analyse the cellular interrelationships of the malignancy. Various maturation compartments with specific phenotypes and proliferative abilities can be recognized. The AML clonogenic cells display specific phenotypes, which may not be representive of the dominant or general AML phenotype. Thus, purging autografts from AML cells may miss the critical precursor cells, unless their phenotype and subsequent removal is especially verified.

REFERENCES

1. Thomas ED, Buckner CD, Clift RA, et al. Marrow transplantation for acute non lymphoblastic leukemia in first remission. N Engl J Med 1979; 301:597–9.
2. Blume KG, Beutler E, Bross KJ, et al. Bone marrow ablation and allogeneic marrow transplantation in acute leukemia. N Engl J Med 1980;302: 1041–6.
3. Powles RL, Clink HM, Bandini G, et al. The place of bone marrow transplantation in acute myelogenous leukemia. Lancet 1980;i:1047–50.
4. Thomas ED, Clift RA, Buckner CD. Marrow transplantation for patients with acute non lymphoblastic leukemia who achieve a first remission. Cancer Treat Rep 1982;66:1463–6.
5. Dicke KA, Spitzer G, Peters L, et al. Autologous bone marrow transplantation in relapsed adult acute leukemia. Lancet 1979;i:514–7.
6. Ishidate M, Aoshima M, Sakurai Y. Population changes of a rat leukemia by different sorts of transplantation. J Natl Cancer Inst 1974;53:773–9.
7. Hagenbeek A. Introduction of BN myelocytic leukemia. Leuk Res 1977;1: 85–90.
8. Harris EB, Hoezler D. Proliferation kinetics of the L5222 leukemia in vivo. Leuk Res 1977;1:93–5.
9. Skipper HE, Schabel FM, Wilcox WS. Experimental evaluation of potential anti-cancer agents. XIII. On the criteria and kinetics associated with "curability" of experimental leukemia. Cancer Chemother Rept 1964;35: 1–111.
10. Touw IP, Löwenberg B. Differentiation of human acute myeloid leukemias following colony formation in vitro detected with monoclonal antibodies. Blood 1984 (submitted).
11. Wouters R, Löwenberg B. On the maturation order of AML cells: a distinction on the basis of self-renewal properties and immunologic phenotypes. Blood 1984;63:684–9.
12. Tax WJM, Willems HW, Kibbelaar MBA, et al. Monoclonal antibodies against human thymocytes and T lymphocytes. In: Peeters H, ed. Protides of the biological fluids. Oxford: Pergamonn Press 29th Colloquium, 1981:701–4.
13. Van der Reyden HJ, Van Rhenen DJ, Lansdorp PM, et al. A comparison of surface marker analysis and FAB classification in acute myeloid leukemia. Blood 1983; 61:433–8.
14. Ferrero D, Pessano S, Pagliardi GL, Rovera G. Induction of differentiation of human myeloid leukemias: surface changes probed with monoclonal antibodies. Blood 1983;61:171–9.
15. Pegoraro L, Abrahm J, Cooper RA, et al. Differentiation of human leukemias in response to 12-0-tetra-decanoylphorbol-13-acetata in vitro. Blood 1980;55:859–62.

DISCUSSION

Moderators: J. van der Wijk, M. Körbling

C.Th. Smit Sibinga (Groningen, The Netherlands):

Dr. James, could you please give some indication as to what percentage of your bone-marrow donors is a blood donor as well?

D.C.O. James (London, U.K.):

I would say about 50% of our donors are also blood donors.

M. Körbling (Heidelberg, FRG):

Do you know how many unrelated bone-marrow transplantations have been performed so far, in the world? More than 50?

D.C.O. James:

No. Certainly not reported. I would imagine that it is on the order of maybe about 20.

M. Körbling:

Dr. Goldman, do you see a real advantage of using blood instead of bone marrow to harvest stem cells? Is there a future for using blood to harvest stem cells? It is of special interest for the Blood Bank, because as you know using a blood cell separator for harvesting peripheral stem cells is a rather easy procedure and cryopreserving such stem cells is not a big deal. I think there is general agreement that peripheral blood stem cells can easily be frozen and cryopreserved for a long time.

J.M. Goldman (London, U.K.):

It is obviously an important question, because if one could collect stem cells from the peripheral blood of a normal individual with a standard leukapheresis procedure, maybe a series of five or ten standard leukapheresis procedures, this would obviate the requirement for a bone-marrow harvest, which would undoubtedly be a benefit. The Seattle Group and the International Bone Marrow Transplant Registry have recently put together the list of complications following bone-marrow harvest*. Although the frequency of the complications is low, the general pattern of the complications is im-

* Bortin MM for the Advisory Committee of the International Bone Marrow Transplant Registry (IBMTR), and Buckner CD for the Seattle Bone Marrow Transplant Team (SMMTT). Major complication of marrow harvesting for transplantation. Exper Hematol 1983;11:916–21.

pressive. There have been cerebral infarctions, pulmonary emboli, cardiac arrests, and even one death of a normal donor. The complications of leukapheresis would be much less.

The question relates to whether stem cells in the peripheral blood of man are adequate to restore hemopoiesis. In animals, we know the answer to that question is "yes". Murine, canine and baboon blood-derived stem cells can all reconstitute hemopoiesis, but in man the evidence is rather scanty. There is no totally convincing example of blood-derived stem cells from normal man reconstituting hemopoiesis. But by extrapolation, one would think that it is possible. It may be just a question of perfecting the technology, rather than that the concept is wrong in principle.

M. Körbling:

I think this is very interesting and it shows that the number required can be achieved. I would like to add two other points: one as related to the allotransplantation situation. For prevention of GvHD, several groups have now undertaken approaches to remove T cells from the bone-marrow graft, for example, using complement mediated cytotoxicity procedures with monoclonal antibodies. Cell suspensions from blood may be disadvantageous in this respect, because the contamination of T-lymphocytes is much greater. This may be a point to keep in mind. Second, as far as autotransplantation is concerned, it would of course be important to see how the contamination of sub-clinical leukemia is. We have no information on this. It may be that the blood would be a very attractive source, but there are no facts on this yet. I agree with you. I think blood stem cells for bone-marrow transplantation should be restricted to autologous transplantations. What about the purging of the stem cell graft? Dr. Löwenberg, do you think that we can separate out the tumor cells?

B. Löwenberg:

As I indicated, I think this approach is not likely to be very promising in the near future. For several reasons, because of the differences between patients. Even if you would establish a generally applicable separation procedure, it is difficult to establish its value, unless you would cure 100% of the patients. One problem is the heterogeneity of the disease and the variability between different patients. In the Rotterdam Symposium on Minimal Residual Disease in Acute Leukemia (Martinus Nijhoff Publishers, 1984), there has been a very interesting suggestion: Why separate out the leukemic cells? In the mouse one can separate out up to 100% purity of normal stem cells. If you would develop a common procedure in which you could select out the pluripotent stem cells, you could use it in every patient. This would be a more profitable approach, also in terms of cell numbers, because the graft is more likely to be enriched for pluripotent stem cells than for subclinical leukemia cells.

W.G. Ho:

Dr. Löwenberg, I wonder how your data regarding the growth characteristics of the circulating stem cells, fit in the context of what we learned from Dr. Glassman in regard to his statement that there are only about 1 or 2% of these circulating stem cells in the blood. This brings up the question that we really do not know for sure whether the stem cell is present in the circulating blood and carries out the same function as in the bone-marrow, even though they may be derived from the same sort of cell. There are probably some differences. There are other groups reporting that the growth characteristics of the circulating stem cells are really not the same as that in the bone marrow*.

Dr. Löwenberg, you said that the purging of the blast cells from remission marrow is going to be a difficult thing. I think we all recognize that, because it is very difficult to control the system once you start to add monoclonal antibodies.

But that brings us to a different story. The fact that you have shown that four patients were in a prolonged remission after autologous transplantation still does not tell us a lot in regard to whether that procedure really is going to be useful for patients with leukemia remission. We are aware of the fact that there are a number of patients with acute leukemia who appear to be surviving in remission after chemotherapy for the induction of remission and who are now five or ten years alive after their initial remission status. I think a point that has to be made is that controlled studies have to be conducted properly before we actually do know what the efficacy of any manipulation is going to be. The correct controls for autologous transplants with unmanipulated bone marrows would be two: One, the natural history of the disease itself, once remission is induced. Secondly, the situation where the marrow that is infused into transplant patients is absolutely clean, like in syngeneic bone-marrow transplant, where the identical twin does not have leukemia and that marrow would not cause graft-versus-host or interstitial pneumonia. We have some data available already from the work of the Seattle Group** and other groups throughout the world in which probably 30 to 50 types of transplants were carried out in that setting. The relapse rate appears to be at least 50%, so we really have to be careful about what the result of untreated autologous marrow will show.

B. Löwenberg:

I think there is no disagreement between us. I would not yet draw any conclusions on the value of autologous transplantation. Nevertheless, if one could show even a 30% disease free survival at the end, it would be at least as good as the best chemotherapy at present; the VAPA-10 protocol for AML continues to show relapses. There is no plateau following chemotherapy.

Dr. Goldman has referred to the J-5 incubations. There are no long-term survivors yet, and there has been a high relapse rate in every recent update. All patients are still in the first year. There is a need of having the unaltered (no tumor cell separation) transplants as controls, in AML as

* Epstein RB, Sarpel SC. Circulating hematopoietic stem cells. In: Gale RP, Fox CF, eds. Biology of bone marrow transplantation. ICN-UCLA Symposia on Molecular and Cellular Biology, vol. 17 New York, Alan R Liss Inc., Academic Press, 1980:405–16.

** Fefer A, Einstein AD, Thomas ED. Bone marrow transplantation for hematologic neoplasia in 16 patients with identical twins. N Engl J Med 1974;290:1389–96.

well as in CML, otherwise there is no way to systematically evaluate any approach of purging.

J.P. Hester:

You answered the question, Dr. Löwenberg. In adult acute leukemia the long-term survival and complete remission are only about 10% of the patients. However, 90% of them are going to relapse. Out of the options for treatment, the effect of chemotherapy reinduction in the second and third remission remains very low. So, autologous transplantation, even with its problems, remains a viable choice.

M. Körbling:

Dr. Goldman, can you give us a short comment on the reconstitutive capacity of blood derived stem cells?

J.M. Goldman:

In relation to man, there really are no important data in the normal situation. There is a study with identical twins reported by McCredie in 1981*. There is also an interesting study reported by Herschko et al. in 1979**, in which a patient with aplastic anemia had a normal identical twin. They tried to induce hemopoietic reconstitution with blood-derived stem cells and failed. They subsequently were successful with marrow-derived stem cells. The study could be criticized on the basis of the relatively small cell numbers used. There is a study reported by Abrams et al.*** in which they tried to achieve hematological reconstitution in a patient undergoing chemotherapy for Ewing's sarcoma, who also had a normal identical twin. Here also, the study was somewhat equivocal. So, using normal man as a source of blood stem cells, on can not really draw firm conclusions.

The real question in Dr. Körbling's mind was whether the data we have for chronic granulocytic leukemia can or cannot legitimately be extrapolated to normal man. At the moment, I do not know the answer to that.

P.C. Das (Groningen, The Netherlands):

Dr. James, with regards to running the Anthony Nolan Unit, how much does it cost? You have to have a collection system for testing, then you have testing and you have a computer in which to feed the data. So, you have three sets of procedures. Could you estimate these procedures and tell us how much it costs to run this unit?

* McCredie KB, Freireich EJ, Hersh EM, Curtis JE, Kaizer H. Early bone marrow recovery after chemotherapy following the transfusion of peripheral blood leukocytes in identical twins. Proc Amer Assoc Cancer Res 1970;11:50.
** Hershko, Gale RP, Ho WG, Cline MJ. Cure of aplastic anemia in paroxysmal nocturnal hemoglobinuria by marrow transfusion from identical twins: failure of peripheral leukocyte transfusion to correct marrow aplasia. Lancet 1979;i:945.
*** Abrams RA, Glaubiger D, Appelbaum FR, Deisseroth AB. Result of attempted hemopoietic reconstitution using isologous peripheral blood mononuclear cells: a case report. Blood 1980;56:516–20.

D.C. James:

Could you just give me the three groups?

P.C. Das:

You have to have a group of donors. You need an administration to know these people's address so that you can organize a collection system. Point two, you need the laboratory HLA typing. Point three, you have to put the data into the computer. Have you any idea how much each "compartment" does cost? The reason why I ask you is that you said that 50% of your donors are blood donors. I presume that 50% of these addresses are available, and they give blood. I presume then that the information is "computerized". Then the costs become slightly different. This is the point I am trying to find out.

D.C.O. James:

I am not sure whether I can answer those questions in that sense. We have not yet been able to compute and get figures of that sort. We have only been able to release certain overall figures, which have really no relationship whatever to the fact that 50% of our donors are also blood donors. When I say they are blood donors that means that they are registered with the National Blood Transfusion Service, so that they give donations of blood to that service on an average of twice a year. These donors also come to us and donate bone marrow, if called up. Of course, the changes are very unlikely in any one case. I do not think it is possible to cost them individually as blood donors. The only figure I can give at the moment is that the cost of HLA typing is £200,000 a year for the unit. This includes every activity that goes on in that unit, research as well. I would break that down to about half the cost going to maintain the register – HLA typing 5,000 people a year. We could say in broad terms that it costs about £20 per person to HLA type any single donor, which is fairly competitive at least in the United Kingdom. I could not go any further at the moment.

C.Th. Smit Sibinga:

Dr. Kootstra, particularly in the last part of your presentation you reported on a system in which, using an extra-corporeal circuit and a membrane oxygenator, kidney preservation will probably be extended tremendously. The question is: What kind of fluids for perfusion do you think are most likely to be used in this ex-vivo situation? Because you will need oxygen to be carried into the organ, do you think of red cells of the recipient, do you want them of donors, or do you think of other sources of oxygen carrying capacity, like fluorocarbons?

G. Kootstra (Maastricht, The Netherlands):

In the experiments we performed, we used blood that was drained right away from the donor dog into the heart-lung machine. The donor dog was anesthetized and bled through a canula into one carotic artery. The whole blood was introduced into the venous reservoir. Within two minutes, we had the kidney in the system and on perfusion. The work of Nizet* from Liège has suggested that this is very important, because if you store blood vasoactive agents will be released into the stored blood. These vasoactive agents cannot be cleared by the kidney and the kidney will go into vasospasm. Of course, the next step in our work will be to look into the effect of red cells, leukocytes and platelets. It will be interesting to see what part of the blood is actually giving the beneficial effect.

M. Körbling:

Dr. Ploeg, I was surprised to notice that 583 kidneys were not transplanted this means 28%. However, you said that there is an increasing demand for donor kidneys.

Is the reason for this not only a question of increase in kidney disease, but also a change in patient selection?

R.J. Ploeg (Leiden, The Netherlands):

I am trying to illustrate that most kidneys which are not used, are not used because of a medical reason before nephrectomy. An additional aspect is refusal of permission. A very important thing seems to be the damage of kidneys.

We noticed an increase in the demand in patients. We need a lot more donors.

As we have seen over the last years an increasing number of patients, the criteria for entering the renal transplant program have widened. The best example is in diabetic patients. This differs from country to country: In Scandinavian countries and in the United States the number of diabetic patients is sometimes even 40% of the whole transplant programme. In other Western European countries, for instance in The Netherlands, it remains up till now rather low, but we do expect this to increase over the coming years.

J.C. Kluin-Neleman (Utrecht, The Netherlands):

Dr. James, how many times can one person donate bone marrow?

D.C.O. James:

The maximum number of times that any donor has given bone marrow in our experience has been twice. I think there have been cases where the same donor has given bone marrow four times – that is, within the family. The transplants had to be repeated on four occasions, so that there is no limit except a logical one: The donor cannot be asked to give bone marrow more than once. We would probably have a limit of two donations for un unrelated donor.

J.C. Kluin-Neleman:

Is there a limit in time-interval between bone-marrow donations?

* Nizet A. The isolated perfused kidney: Possibilities, limitations and results. Ed Review, Kidney Int. 1975;7:1.

D.C.O. James:

The interval required before bone marrow is regenerated adequately is, I suppose on the order of two months. I think that after that they could give a second donation.

J.M. Goldman:

In actual fact it is not a practical problem at all. We found it necessary to use three donors on more than one occasion in the past four years. In each case we were unimpressed by the quality of engraftment after the first donation and we asked the donor to repeat the procedure roughly four weeks later. We got good engraftment on each of the second occasions. You see, if you imagine that you are removing just about 1% of the donor's marrow in a routine harvest, there is quite a large reserve for the donor. I have been talking about donors related to the patient and therefore I would share Dr. James' feeling that when you are dealing with an unrelated donor you should be more circumspect in your efforts to protect that person. But, from a physiological standpoint, you could collect more than once quite safely.

IV. SPECIFIC ORGAN TRANSPLANTATION

KIDNEY TRANSPLANTATION - CURRENT PERSPECTIVE

R.F.M. Wood

The technique of renal transplantation, with the creation of an extra-peritoneal pouch in the groin and anastomosis of the renal artery and vein to the iliac vessels, has remained standard practice since it was devised in the 1950s. In experienced centres the rate of early technical complications is extremely low. Late complications include renal artery stenosis and ureteric stricture with the development of hydronephrosis. Both these problems are amenable to surgical correction and encouraging results have been reported with Gruntzig Balloon Dilatation for renal artery stenosis (1).

The cocktail of azathioprine and prednisolone was developed as standard immunosuppressive therapy almost 20 years ago. It is disappointing that despite a large research effort few of the many compounds that are active in vitro or in experimental animals have proved to be effective in man. The increased susceptibility to infection caused by the current immunosuppressive therapy is a major cause of morbidity in renal transplant patients and viral infections, especially cytomegalovirus, remain a significant problem. However, the figures from the European Dialysis and Transplant Association show that there has been a progressive reduction in mortality over the past 15 years. One year patient survival in cadaver graft recipients in 1969 was just over 70%, by 1979 the figure had improved to over 80%. Between 1979 and 1982 the one year patient survival for recipients between the ages of 15 and 44 was in excess of 90%. Even with careful selection and management between a quarter and a third of cadaver grafts will be lost to rejection during the first year. Research effort is therefore concentrated on improving tissue matching and investigating methods of immunosuppression or immune regulation that will have a more specific action on the pathways responsible for sensitization and the generation of effector cells, without the unwanted side effects of current therapy.

CYTOTOXIC ANTIBODIES

Cytotoxic antibodies which can cause hyperacute rejection, may be present in the sera of potential recipients as a result of pregnancy, blood transfusion or a previous failed graft. Hyperacute rejection is irreversible and characterized by destruction of the vascular endothelium of the transplanted kidney, due to activation of both the complement and coagulation pathways. After revascularisation the kidney rapidly becomes blue and flaccid due to blockage of the glomerular capillaries by platelet thrombi. The detection of cytotoxic antibodies in a pre-transplant cross-match test is a routine procedure in clinical transplantation and a positive result has been regarded as an absolute contraindication to operation. Antibodies occur more frequently than was previously recognized and serum samples collected after blood transfusion, at the time of acute rejection and following graft nephrectomy will frequently have significant levels of antibody activity when tested against a panel of normal lymphocytes (2). In any long established transplant unit routine screening for cytotoxic antibodies will reveal the presence of a sizeable group of "highly sensitized" patients. These patients may repeatedly have positive cross-match against apparently suitable donors and often come to be regarded as untransplantable because of the risks of hyperacute rejection. However, the development of more sophisticated analyses of the cross-match test have demonstrated that not all these antibodies are liable to cause hyperacute rejection. The work of Ting (3,4) has shown that many patients have auto-antibodies which, although causing a cytotoxic reaction with donor T and B lymphocytes in vitro will not cause hyperacute rejection in vivo. The presence of these auto-antibodies can be detected by screening the sera against a panel of B lymphocytes from patients with chronic lymphatic leukemia (CLL). These CLL cells express HLA-A, -B, -C and -DR antigens on their surface and a positive reaction to CLL cells indicates the presence of broadly reactive cytotoxic antibody. However, the serum of patients who have auto-antibodies will not react with CLL cells. The results of transplantation in Oxford in patients with positive cross-matches due to auto-reactive antibodies are shown in Figure 1. There is no difference in graft survival between the patients who were cross-match negative and those who had either a postive B cell cross-match or a positive B + T cell cross-match to auto-reactive antibodies.

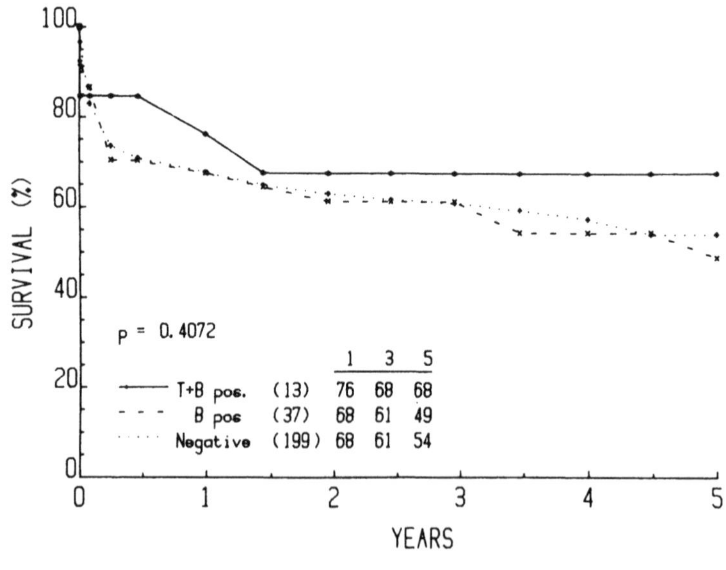

Figure 1. Graft survival in cross-match negative patients in Oxford compared to graft survival with either a positive B cell cross-match or a positive B + T cell cross-match due to auto-antibodies.

Despite the encouraging results of transplantation in patients with autoantibodies there remains the problem of transplantation in patients with broadly reactive antibodies, cytotoxic for over 90% of panel lymphocytes. Attempts are being made in some centres to deplete the patients of circulating antibody by plasmapheresis and to block further antibody production by the use of immunosuppression. However, the effectiveness of this policy in preventing hyperacute rejection remains to be established.

TISSUE TYPING

In Europe matching for HLA-A and B locus antigens has been used as the basis of tissue matching and organ sharing for the past 15 years. However, the value of HLA-A, B matching in transplantation remains controversial. The London Transplant Group reporting the results of 889 transplants performed between 1969 and 1979 show a highly significant influence of A and B matching on graft survival (5). However, the results from large collective series, such as the 2014 cases reported in 1982 by Opelz and Terasaki (6) have failed to show any correlation between graft survival and HLA-A and -B locus matching. The D region situated closer to the centromere of chromosome 6 than the HLA-A and -B loci has been known to have an important influence on the outcome of transplantation. Initially D locus identity was established by mixed lymphocyte culture over 5 days and was therefore only practicable in live donor transplantation. The discovery of D locus antigens on the surface of B lymphocytes paved the way for a serological determination of D locus compatibility-DR matching (7). Since there is a single DR locus, only two matches are required for complete identity and it has been calculated that with a pool size of 300 there is a 95% chance of obtaining a DR compatible recipient for any kidney on offer. The results of DR matching in Oxford are shown in Figure 2 with 79% one year graft survival in patients receiving kidneys with no DR mis-matches.

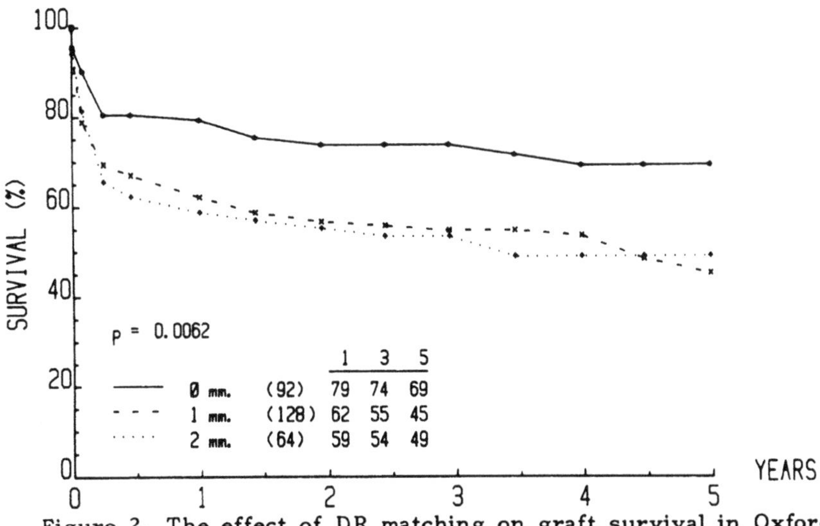

Figure 2. The effect of DR matching on graft survival in Oxford.

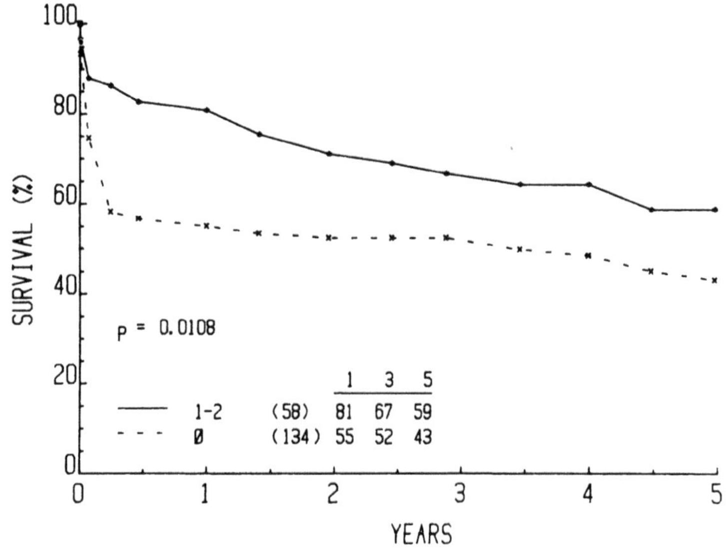

Figure 3. The effect of 1 to 2 transfusions on graft survival in Oxford.

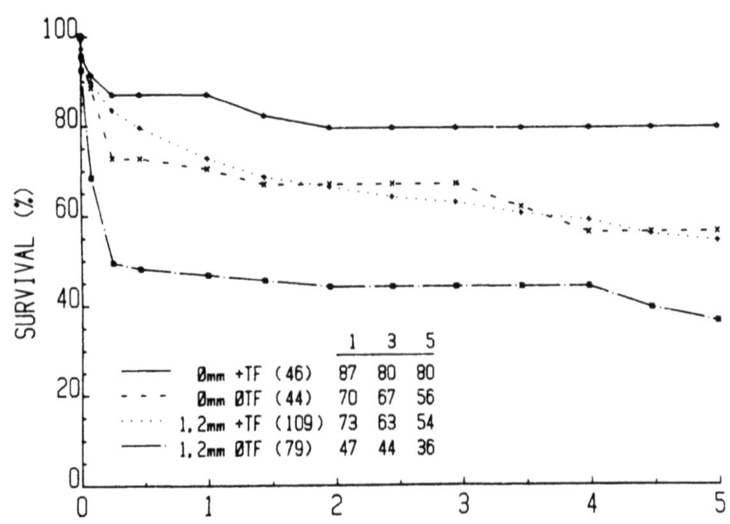

Figure 4. The additive effect of DR matching and blood transfusion in the Oxford Series.

This was significantly better (p=0.006) than the 61% one year graft survival in patients whose transplants were mis-matched for DR. Further information on the value of DR matching in large series is still awaited. However, the pooled results from North America already show a statistically significant advantage for DR matched versus DR mis-matched donor recipient combinations (6).

Increasing knowledge of the major histocompatibility system will undoubtedly be acquired during the next few years. In some ways this additional information may only complicate the practical problem of matching donors and recipients. However, for patients with a given tissue type it may be possible in future to identify specificities to which they will have a strong response and therefore to be able to map out a series of "acceptable" donor tissue-types for each individual recipient.

BLOOD TRANSFUSION AND ALLOGRAFT ENHANCEMENT

During the 1960s the majority of patients receiving kidney transplants had been polytransfused while on dialysis. It was recognized that transfusion caused in increased incidence of cytotoxic antibody formation and it was felt that transplant results would probably be better in non-sensitized patients who had never been transfused. Improvements in dialysis coupled with concern about the risks of hepatitis led to a reduction in blood transfusion and by the early 1970s there was a large pool of dialysis patients who had never been transfused. It soon became apparent that these non-transfused individuals faired poorly after transplantation and that unplanned blood transfusion had a beneficial effect on allograft survival (8–10). Experience in Oxford (Fig. 3) has shown that one year graft survival after only one or two units of blood is significantly better at 81%, than the 55% one year graft survival in non-transfused patients. DR matching and blood transfusion appear to have an additive effect on graft survival (Fig. 4). In addition to its proven benefit on cadaver allograft survival blood transfusion can be used to improve results of mis-matched live donor transplants. Salvatierra et al. (11) have reported a one year graft survival rate of 94% in 101 patients transplanted with a one-haplotype matched kidney after donor specific transfusion.

Although many units now adopt a policy of deliberate transfusion, concern has been expressed that a liberal transfusion policy will lead to an increasing number of highly sensitized patients (12). There is also no general agreement on a transfusion protocol which will provide enhancement with a minimal incidence of sensitization. Primate experiments have suggested that platelet transfusions may be effective in producing enhancement without the risks of inducing cytotoxic antibody formation (13) but these observations have yet to be confirmed in human transplantation.

Despite the potency of blood transfusion in improving transplant survival the underlying mechanism is still unclear. It has been proposed that suppressor cells (14) may be involved or that blood transfusions cause a transient impairment of macrophage activity (15). More recently it has been demonstrated that blood transfusion induces the formation of anti-idiotypic antibodies and it is postulated that these antibodies are responsible for allograft enhancement (16). If the factors in the blood which are responsible for the transfusion effect could be clearly defined graft survival could be improved and the potential complications of elective transfusion avoided.

IMMUNOSUPPRESSION

"Low dose" steroids

Long-term steroid immunosuppression has had distressing side-effects in renal transplant patients. Cushingoid facies, hypertension, diabetes mellitus, skin changes and avascular necrosis of bone are common problems causing significant morbidity. The "low dose" steroid regime popularized by McGeown in Belfast (17) has produced a considerable reduction in steroid associated problems. Initial protocols for steroid immunosuppression utilized doses of prednisolone of up to 200 mg per day around the time of transplantation with the dose slowly tapered over several months. In the Belfast regime patients receive only 20 mg of prednisolone per day for the first six months after operation followed by a gradual reduction to the long-term maintenance level of 10 mg per day. The benefit of this regimen has now been confirmed by a number of other units (18,19).

Cyclosporin A (CyA)

CyA is the most significant new immunosuppressive drug to have been discovered since the development of the immunosuppressive cocktail of azathioprine and prednisolone in the 1960s (20). It is produced as a metabolite by the soil fungus Tolypocladium Inflatum Gams. Early laboratory research demonstrated that CyA was particularly potent in suppressing the initial response of the immune system to foreign antigen. It is postulated that CyA

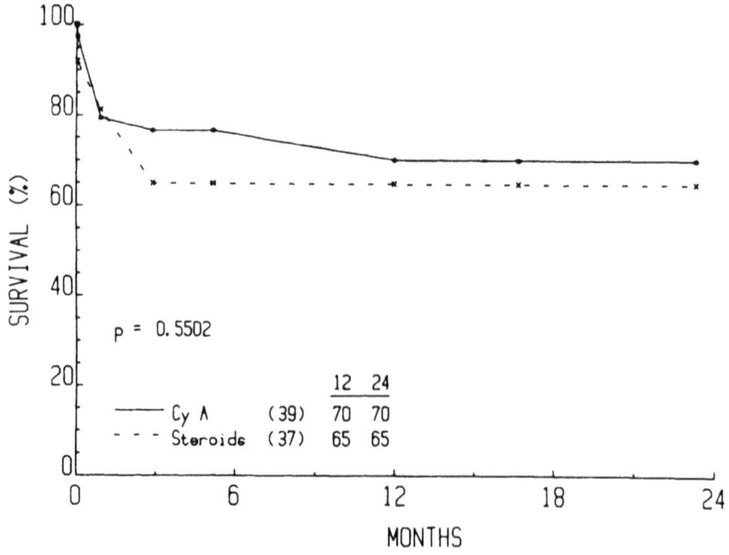

Figure 5. Current graft survival in the Oxford trial of Cyclosporin A (CyA). The control group received azathioprine and prednisolone (AP) from the time of transplantation. In the CyA group the drug was given as the sole form of immunosuppression for the first three months with conversion to AP at 90 days.

affects the synthetic machinery of the cell, blocking the antigen derived signal required to stimulate the production of cytotoxic T cells.

In early clinical studies although the drug appeared to be effective in preventing rejection there were a number of cases of lymphoma due to combining CyA with large doses of other immunosuppressives (21). Subsequent multicentre trials in Canada and Europe have shown that CyA produces a significant improvement in one year graft survival. In the European trial, involving 232 patients, one year graft survival in the group treated with CyA was 73% compared 53% one year graft survival in the control group treated with azathioprine and prednisolone (22). CyA is undoubtedly both nephrotoxic and hepatotoxic and these complications can cause difficult management problems. In the Oxford trial of CyA patients have been converted from CyA to azathioprine and prednisolone three months after transplantation in an attempt to avoid long-term side effects (23). The CyA treated patients have improved graft survival compared to patients on conventional therapy from the time of transplantation (Fig. 5) and serum creatinine rapidly returns to normal following conversion (Table I).

Table I. Serum creatinine (SCr) changes following conversion from Cyclosporin A alone to azathioprine and prednisolone (28 patients).

	Conversion (C)	C + 1/52	C + 1/12	C + 3/12
Mean serum creatinine (μmol/l ± SD)	242 ± 89	167 ± 52	131 ± 34	126 ± 38
% fall in mean SCr		31	46	48
Range	(141–489)	(104–331)	(72–184)	(67–194)
Significance of fall in serum creatinine		p=0.001	p=0.01	p=0.62

Monoclonal antibodies

Reagents are now available with reactivity againts determinants on lymphocyte subpopulations and preliminary clinical trials have been carried out where pan T cell monoclonals have been used to treat acute rejection. The antibodies employed, OKT3 and anti-T12, have been shown to be effective in reversing rejection although the development of antibodies to mouse immunoglobulins precludes their use on a long-term basis.

Alternative approaches to immunosuppression

Local irradiation of an enlarged, rejecting graft will cause dramatic shrinkage but the beneficial effect is probably counterbalanced by radiation damage to the tubules and glomeruli. Total lymphoid irradiation (TLI) with the protocol development for the treatment of Hodgkins disease has been suggested for use in highly sensitized patients but clinical results have been disappointing with significant complications. Thoracic duct drainage of lymph with centrifugation and retransfusion of supernatant plasma is an effective means of removing lymphocytes during the immediate post-operative period (24). However, it is difficult to maintain drainage on a long-term basis and the procedure is standard practice in only a few units. Lymphoid depletion by splenectomy remains controversial in view of the risks of infection but a controlled trial from Minneapolis has shown that it conveys a significant benefit to patients treated with ALG (25).

IMMUNOLOGICAL MONITORING

A wide variety of in vitro immunological tests have been used in an attempt to diagnose rejection before there is an alteration in biochemical parameters (26). However, techniques detecting changes in lymphocyte and antibody activity in the peripheral blood, although providing valuable information on the mechanism of rejection, have so far failed to gain acceptance in the routine management of transplant patients. Renewed interest in monitoring has been stimulated by the availability of monoclonal antibodies which enable T lymphocyte subpopulations, B cells and monocytes/macrophages to be separately identified. Several groups have reported on the ratio of helper/inducer to suppressor/cytotoxic T lymphocytes in the peripheral blood of transplant patients. This ratio does not appear to be helpful in predicting rejection (27). However, patients with a ratio of less than 1.0 have been found to have a high instance of viral infection (28). Fine-needle aspiration biopsy has become an established method for monitoring cellular changes within the graft (29). The cytological preparations can be stained with conventional hematological stains but more detailed information can be obtained by using immunoperoxidase staining with monoclonal antibodies to obtain an accurate picture of the subpopulations of infiltrating lymphocytes (30). Early rejection is characterized by blast cell infiltration with the majority of cells having the suppressor/cytotoxic T8 phenotype. In severe rejection increasing numbers of monocytes and tissue macrophages are identified indicating marked tissue destruction.

The development of additional forms of immunosuppressive treatment create the problem of deciding which form of therapy to use in the individual patient. Ideally it should be possible, using monitoring techniques, to identify different patterns of rejection with the possibility of tailoring the immunosuppressive regimen to the patients's individual requirements.

REFERENCES

1. Mollenkopf F, Matas A, Veith FJ. Percutaneous transluminal angioplasty for transplant renal artery stenosis. Transplant Proc 1983;15:1089–91.
2. Morris PJ, Ting A. The cross-match in renal transplantation. Tissue Antigens 1981;17:75–82.
3. Ting A, Morris PJ. Renal transplantation and B-cell cross-matches with autoantibodies and alloantibodies. Lancet 1977;ii:1095–7.
4. Ting A, Morris PJ. Reactivity of autolymphocytotoxic antibodies from dialysis patients with lymphocytes from chronic lymphocytic leukemia (CLL) patients. Transplantation 1978;25:31–3.
5. Festenstein H, Sachs JA, Butterfield K, Yeatman N, Holmes J. Collaborative scheme for tissue typing and matching in renal transplantation. XI. Role of HLA-A, B, DR and D matching and other factors on 899 cadaver kidney grafts. Transplant Proc 1981;13:934–7.

6. Opelz G, Terasaki PI. International study of histocompatibility in renal transplantation. Transplantation 1982;33:87–95.
7. Bodmer WF, Batchelor JR, Bodmer JG, Festenstein H, Morris PJ, eds. Histocompatibility testing (Report of the 7th International Histocompatibility Workshop and Conference, Oxford) Copenhagen: Munsgaard, 1977.
8. Opelz G, Sengar DPS, Mickey MR, Terasaki PI. Effect of blood transfusions on subsequent kidney transplants. Transplant Proc 1973;5:253–9.
9. Van Es AA, Balner H. Effect of pretransplant transfusions on kidney allograft survival. Transplant Proc 1979;11:127–37.
10. Opelz G, Terasaki PI. Dominant effect of transfusions on kidney allograft survival. Transplantation 1980;29:153–8.
11. Salvatierra JR, Vincenti W, Amend Jr M, et al. Four-year experience with donor-specific blood transfusions. Transplant Proc 1983;15:924–31.
12. Editorial. Blood transfusions and renal transplantation. Lancet 1978; ii:193–4.
13. Borleffs JCC, Neuhaus P, Van Rood JJ, Balner H. Platelet transfusion improve kidney allograft survival in Rhesus monkeys without inducing cytotoxic antibodies. Lancet 1982;i:1117–8.
14. Van Rood JJ, Balner H, Morris PJ. Blood transfusion and transplantation. Transplantation 1978;26:275–7.
15. Keown PA, Descamps B. Improved renal allograft survival after blood transfusions: a non-specific erythrocyte-mediated immuno-regulatory process? Lancet 1979;i:20–2.
16. Singal DP, Fagnilli L, Joseph S. Blood transfusions induce anti-idiotypic antibodies in renal transplant patients. Transplant Proc 1983;15: 1005–8.
17. McGeown MG, Kennedy JA, Loughridge WGG, et al. One hundred transplants in the Belfast City Hospital. Lancet 1977;ii:648–51.
18. Morris PJ, Chan L, French ME, Ting A. Low dose oral prednisolone in renal transplantation. Lancet 1982;i:525–7.
19. Salaman JR, Griffin PJA, Price K. High or low dose steroids for immunosuppression. Transplant Proc 1983;15:1086–8.
20. Morris PJ. Cyclosporin A. Transplantation 1982;32:349–54.
21. Calne RY, Rolles K, White DJG, et al. Cyclosporin A initially as the only immunosuppressant in 34 recipients of cadaveric organs: 32 kidneys, 2 pancreases and 2 livers. Lancet 1979;ii:1033–6.
22. European Multicentre Trial. Cyclosporin A as sole immunosuppressive agent in recipients of kidney allografts from cadaver donors. Lancet 1982;ii:57–60.
23. Morris PJ, French ME, Dunnill MS, et al. A controlled trial of Cyclosporine in renal transplantation with conversion to azathioprine and prednisolone after 3 months. Transplantation 1983;36:273–7.
24. Frankkson C, Lundgen G, Magnusson G, Ringden, O. Drainage of thoracic duct lymph in renal transplant patients. Transplantation 1976;21:133–40.
25. Fryd DS, Sutherland DER, Simmons RL, Ferguson RM, Kjellstand CM, Najarian JS. Results of a prospective randomized study on the effect of splenectomy in renal transplant patients. Transplant Proc 1981;13:48–59.
26. Wood RFM. Immunological monitoring after renal transplantation. In: Morris PJ, ed. Kidney transplantation, principles and practice. London, Orlando, New York Grune & Straffon, 2nd edition 1984.
27. Carter NP, Cullen PR, Thompson JF, Bewick ALT, Wood RFM, Morris PJ. Monitoring lymphocyte subpopulations in renal allograft recipients. Transplant Proc 1983;15:1157–9.

28. Chatenoud L, Chkoff N, Kreis H, Bach JF. Correlation between immunoregulatory T-cell imbalances and renal allograft outcome. Transplant Proc 1983;15:1184–5.
29. Hayry P, von Willebrand E. Cytologic evaluation of in situ inflammatory response of rejection in human renal transplantation. Transplant Proc 1981;13:81–3.
30. Wood RFM, Bolton EM, Thompson JF, Morris PJ. Monoclonal antibodies and fine needle aspiration cytology in detecting renal allograft rejection. Lancet 1982;ii:278.

PRESENT STATUS OF CLINICAL LIVER TRANSPLANTATION BASED ON A REVIEW OF 5 CENTRES: PITTSBURGH, CAMBRIDGE, HANNOVER, INNSBRUCK AND GRONINGEN

R.A.F. Krom

From 1963–1983 555 liver transplantations have been performed (Table I). A total of 155 patients were alive in 1983; 81 patients survived more than one year, 23 more than 5 years and 5 even beyond 10 years (Table II). The actuarial one year survival was 35%. The results of more recent years are further improving to 60 and 70% (1).

Table I.

Results until 1983		Number of liver transplantations		Alive
Denver	1963	184	293	89
Pittsburg	1980	109		
Cambridge/KCH	1968		138	24
Hannover	1975		75	20
Paris	1978		11	1
Innsbruck	1978		9	4
Groningen	1979		26	16
1963–1983			555	155

Table II.

Alive 1983	Total	1 year	5 years	10 years
Pittsburgh	89	45	18	5
Cambridge/KCH	24	16	4	-
Hannover	20	10	1	-
Paris	1	1	-	-
Innsbruck	4	2	-	-
Groningen	16	7	-	-
Total	155	81	23	5

PRIMARY DIAGNOSIS (Table III)

The three most common diagnoses for which liver transplantation has been performed are primary liver tumor, cirrhosis and biliary atresia. The most frequent other diagnoses are antitrypsin deficiency and Budd-Chiari syndrome.

Table III. Total number liver transplantations that have been performed for the three most frequent indications (1963–1983).

	Primary liver tumor	Cirrhosis	Biliary atresia
Pittsburgh*	27	125	62
Cambridge/KCH	49	61	2
Hannover	38	20	8
Innsbruck	6	3	-
Groningen	1	20	-
Total until 1983	121	229	72

* Until May 1982.

LIVER TUMOR

Until 1983 121 patients with a primary liver tumor have been treated with liver transplantation. Only 4 of all patients who have been transplanted in Denver/Pittsburgh until 1982 for liver tumor survived one year. The majority of the 11 patients that survived the operative procedure died with tumor recurrence.

Also in Cambridge only 10 out of 25 patients survived one year, but 6 of these patients died later with tumor recurrence (2,3).

In Hannover ± 50% of the patients has been transplanted for primary liver tumor. The results are disappointing as ± 80% of the patients died due to recurrent disease within the first and second year after liver transplantation.

However, all centres have individual long-term survivors, emphasizing the need of meticulous preoperative screening for extrahepatic metastases, and perhaps for the histological type of liver tumor.

CIRRHOSIS

A total of 229 patients have been transplanted for end-stage liver cirrhosis until 1983. The majority suffered from chronic active cirrhosis (120 patients) and from primary biliary cirrhosis (48 patients). Out of 61 patients with a variety of other cirrhotic liver disease, 19 were known to have alcoholic liver cirrhosis.

Until 1980 the results were moderate, reflected by a one-year survival of ± 30%. Since then, however, the results have improved regarding the reported one-year survival rates of 60–70%.

Principally patients whith end-stage liver cirrhosis are ideal candidates for liver transplantation, because they lack the risk of rapid recurrence of primary disease as in patients with livertumor. However, the often poor physical condition makes liver transplantation a risky surgical procedure with substantial operative mortality. An important problem is the coagulation abnormalities, intrinsic to the deterioration of liver function, with subsequent massive peroperative bloodloss. Many of these patients died postoperatively due to multi organ failure.

Obviously, there are two ways to approach these problems. Firstly it may be necessary to exclude patients whose liver function has been deteriorated too far. Groningen evaluated the preoperative data of the patients in relation to bloodloss. This relation was significantly positive regarding parameters belonging to the hepatorenal syndrome and to synthetic liverfunction, as coagulation factors and antithrombin III, and albumen (3).

According to these data it might be possible to detect these poor risk patients, and to improve patient selection. Secondly one can search for better surgical techniques and ways to normalize the peroperative coagulation status or to reduce the peroperative bloodloss. Pittsburgh introduced recently the porto-caval axillary venous bypass (4), in order to decrease the portal hypertension and to restore the systemic circulation during the anhepatic period. Bloodloss and hemodynamics improved markedly by this procedure.

Previously Cambridge used an arteriovenous bypass to diminish the venous trapping of the blood and to improve the arterial blood pressure. Although success has been mentioned this procedure has not been used routinely. Most centres started to use an autotransfusion system. Coagulation prevention by heparin and citrate both were used.

BILIARY ATRESIA

Only Denver/Pittsburgh has a major experience in pediatric liver transplantation. More than 50% of the children suffered from biliary atresia, but also patients with congenital metabolic diseases, as α_1-antitrypsin deficiency, Wilson's disease and glycogen storage disease, were transplanted.

The results of pediatric liver transplantation from 1963 through 1979 were somewhat better than for adults, but improved markedly since then (1). Very likely cyclosporin A contributed to this improvement of the one-year survival from 38% to 70%, although in the new set up in Pittsburgh the cooperation with the pediatricians has played an important role. In the other centres children have been transplanted only occasionally. Lack of suitable donors and feelings about the moral justification of liver transplantation in children has limited the total number. It can be expected that with the increased life expectancy and the diminished need for the use of prednisone with cyclosporin A the pediatricians will consider liver transplantation more frequently in the future.

LONG-TERM SURVIVING PATIENTS

At the beginning of 1983 155 patients were reported to be alive, of them 109 have survived more than one year and 28 longer than 5 years. Five patients live already more than 10 years beyond liver transplantation. Most of the long-term survivors are well-rehabilitated and participate in daily life by having a full time job or taking care for home and family.

A number of problems remains: The delayed growth of transplanted children, especially of those treated with corticosteroids can lead to emotional problems, while osteoporosis in the elderly PBC patients may lead to a significant shortening of statue. The use of cyclosporin A might improve these complications, but might introduce others, like chronic nephrotoxicity. The effect of long-term immunosuppression on development of tumors de novo is not really known, although the incidence is increased. Presently, the life expectance with a transplanted liver is totally unknown, but the increasing number of long-term survivors and the good quality of life makes liver transplantation worthwhile.

FUTURE OF LIVER TRANSPLANTATION

The improving results of liver transplantation have created hope for many otherwise doomed liver diseased patients. In many medical centres around the world renewed interest has arisen and a start of a liver transplantation program is being considered. In order to determine the present status of liver transplantation in relation to clinical application and research the National Institute of Health organized a consensus development conference in June 1983 (5). The members of the panel came to the following conclusion:

> "After extensive review and consideration of all available data, this panel concludes that liver transplantation is a therapeutic modality for end-stage liver disease that deserves broader application. However, in order for liver transplantation to gain its full therapeutic potential, the indications for and results of the procedure must be the object of comprehensive, coordinated, and ongoing evaluation in the years ahead. This can best be achieved by expansion of this technology to a limited number of centers where performance of liver transplantation can be carried out under optimal conditions."

This conclusion might be the best guide for the next era of liver transplantation.

REFERENCES

1. Starzl TE, Iwatsuki S, Van Thiel DH, et al. Evolution in liver transplantation. Hepatology 1982;2:614–36.
2. Calne RY. Liver transplantation for liver cancer. World J Surg 1982;6:76–80.
3. Iwatsuki S, Klintmalm GBG, Starzl TE. Total hepatectomy and liver replacement (Orthotopic liver transplantation) for primary hepatic malignancy. World J Surg 1982;6:81–5.

4. Krom RAF, Gips CH, Houthoff HJ, et al. Orthotopic liver transplantation in Groningen (The Netherlands 1979–1983). Hepatology 1984;3 (suppl): 61–5.
5. Summary of the Consensus Development Conference in Liver Transplantation. National Institute of Health 1983;4 no. 7.

ALLOGENEIC BONE MARROW TRANSPLANTATION*

W.G. Ho, D.J. Winston, R.E. Champlin, S.A. Feig, R.P. Gale

INTRODUCTION

Transplantation of allogeneic bone marrow is increasingly utlized as a modality of treatment for aplastic anemia and leukemia. Patients with these disorders are usually immunocompetent and are able to reject grafts. It is therefore necessary to immunosuppress these patients in preparation for transplantation from donors other than genetically identical twins.

In general, most pretransplant conditioning regimens in patients with aplastic anemia and leukemia utilize high dose cyclophosphamide alone or in combination with total body irradiation (1,2). After administration of the conditioning regimen, the transplant is carried out by intravenous infusion of $1\text{-}9 \times 10^8$ bone marrow cells per kilogram. Engraftment usually occurs over two to four weeks. In a successful transplant donor type hematopoiesis can be demonstrated by detailed cytogenetic and gene marker studies (3). Following engraftment, graft-versus-host disease (GvHD) and interstitial pneumonia are the major complications that limit the short term success of the treatment.

GvHD results from the immunological reaction of donor T lymphocytes against recipient tissues (4,5). The disease is characterized clinically by necrotic lesions in lymphatic tissues, skin, gastrointestinal tract and liver. Clinical and pathological features of GvHD have been reviewed elsewhere (6,7). Acute GvHD develops in 25% to 75% of recipients of allogeneic marrow transplants. Moderate to severe forms of GvHD occur in approximately 25% of patients and is fatal in half of the cases.

Approaches to prevent GvHD have relied on the use of methotrexate, given intermittently for three months following transplantation. Patients who develop acute GvHD are treated with corticosteroids, antithymocyte globulin or cyclosporin A. These agents can favourably influence the clinical features of GvHD, but probably do not improve survival (8,9). Recent studies suggest that cyclosporin A may be superior to methotrexate in the prevention of GvHD (10).

Innovative approaches to prevent GvHD include the removal of mature T cells from the donor marrow prior to transplantation, either by physical or immunological methods (11). The efficacy of such approaches still remains to be confirmed by appropriate clinical trials.

* Supported by grants CA-23175, from the National Cancer Institute and by grant RR-865 from the Public Health Service. Dr. Champlin is a recipient of a New Investigator Research Award, National Institute of Arthritis, Diabetes and Kidney Disease. Dr. Gale is the Meyerhoff Visiting Scientist of the Weizmann Institute of Science.

Interstitial pneumonia occurs in 25% to 75% of transplant recipients (12). Approximately 50% of cases are associated with cytomegalovirus (CMV) infection. Other pathogens such as adenovirus, Echo virus, respiratory syncytial virus, herpes zoster varicellosus, and Pneumocystis carinii are occasionally implicated (13,14). Numerous factors are involved in the development of interstitial pneumonia and these include exogenous CMV infection, probably via blood transfusions; activation of latent endogenous CMV infections; drug or radiation damage to the lung; GvHD; and post-transplant immunodeficiency.

CMV remains the main pathogen associated with interstitial pneumonia. Attempts to treat established CMV infections with adenosine arabinoside, acyclovir, interferon or combinations of these agents have not been successful (15–19). Attention is therefore currently focussed on the prevention of CMV infection rather than on treatment. Studies of passive immunization by means of CMV antibody preparations appear encouraging (20–22). Exclusive use of CMV seronegative blood components in the transfusion support of transplant recipients may also be useful, since this approach appears effective in other immunocompromised patients (23).

APLASTIC ANEMIA

Patients with aplastic anemia have an extremely poor prognosis with median survival of 3 to 6 months (24). Appropriate therapy consists of transfusion support and control of infections. These interventions treat the symptoms or complications of the disease rather than the disease itself. Therapeutic modalities aimed at correcting the aplasia have included treatment with corticosteroids, androgens, etiocholanolone and lithium. Controlled clinical trials of these agents have shown little evidence of benefit in aplastic anemia (25). A recent trial with antithymocyte globulin indicates that this form of immunosuppressive therapy may be effective in 50% of patients and offers an alternative to bone marrow transplantation, especially for those patients with no suitable HLA matched donor (26).

Most cases of aplastic anemia are believed to be related to a lack of hematopoietic stem cells and replacement of these cells from a histocompatible donor represents a rational approach. Bone marrow transplantation is therefore increasingly used to treat aplastic anemia in patients with an appropriate donor. Several reviews of the efficacy of this approach have been published. Disease free survival rates range from 25% to 74% (27,28). Recent studies indicate survival of greater than 50% in selected patients; survival of younger patients and previously non-transfused patients is superior in most series (29). Unfortunately, few patients are referred for marrow transplantation before receiving transfusions.

Apart from GvHD and interstitial pneumonia, graft rejection is a major problem following transplantation for aplastic anemia. Graft rejection occurs in 25% to 60% of recipients of allogeneic transplants conditioned with cyclophosphamide (200 mg/kg) alone. This problem is more common in patients transfused prior to transplantation (29). Experimental data suggest that graft rejection may be due to sensitization to minor histocompatibility antigens induced by blood product transfusion (30). However, other studies have failed to show a relationship between prior transfusion and graft rejection (31,32). Other mechanisms are probably involved, since graft rejection also occurs in non-transfused patients, as well as in genetically identical monozygotic twin transplants.

Since those patients at high risk for graft rejection cannot be accurately identified pretransplant, approaches to this problem have been directed towards development of conditioning regimens associated with low rates of graft rejection. These have included more intensive chemotherapy, fractionated total body irradiation or total lymphoid irradiation (33,34). Our approach has been to add low doses of total body irradiation to cyclophosphamide (35). This regimen was designed to decrease the risk of graft rejection without increasing the incidence of GvHD or interstitial pneumonia. Two year actuarial survival was 62% and graft rejection was observed in only 1 out of 46 patients.

In summary, for younger patients with aplastic anemia, allogeneic marrow transplantation remains the treatment of choice. Ideally, transplantation should be carried out before transfusions are required. Since most patients require transfusions before transplantation the risk of graft rejection can be decreased and the achievement of excellent transplant results can be obtained, with a conditioning regimen consisting of cylcophosphamide and low dose total body irradiation. For older patients and those without suitably matched donors, alternate forms of therapy such as antithymocyte globulin may prove to be more beneficial.

ACUTE LEUKEMIA

Despite substantial progress in the treatment of leukemia, few patients are cured by conventional therapy. Bone marrow transplantation has therefore been applied in attempt to achieve a cure. Allogeneic marrow transplants in patients with resistant acute leukemia result in a low success rate with actuarial survival of less than 10%. Resistant leukemia is the main cause of treatment failure, followed by GvHD and interstitial pneumonia. Attempts to improve survival by the development of more intensive conditioning regimens to combat resistant leukemia have led to a high incidence of drug and radiation related toxicity and infections. The alternative approach has been to transplant patients in remission.

In acute lymphoblastic leukemia (ALL), the median survival of patients who relapse while receiving maintenance chemotherapy is 6 months and less than 5% survive to two years. Patients who relapse after completing maintenance chemotherapy have a better prognosis with a median survival of 2 years. Results of transplantation in patients with ALL transplanted in second or later remission indicate an actuarial remission rate of 50% with 35% survival at 2 years (36). Survival of transplant patients is clearly superior to survival of patients who are treated with further conventional therapy after relapse while on maintenance chemotherapy.

Data comparing survival of patients transplanted with survival of those who receive conventional chemotherapy for relapse occurring off maintenance chemotherapy indicate a high early mortality in the transplant group. Survival of the two groups is comparable after 2 years. At present it is still unclear whether transplantation has an advantage when carried out in patients who relapse off maintenance chemotherapy. It is also discouraging that the relapse rate exceeds 50% despite transplantation in second remission. It may therefore be reasonable to consider transplantation for those patients with poor prognostic ALL in first remission, such as age 7 years, or T & B cell type ALL.

In acute myelogenous leukemia (AML), there has been a marked development of chemotherapeutic regimens capable of inducing remission in 65% to 80% of patients, with long term survival of 20%. Recent reports indicate that with intensive consolidation chemotherapy after remission, the disease free survival may approach 45% (37).

The results obtained in patients with AML transplanted in first remission are encouraging. The actuarial relapse rate appears to be only 20% at 2 years with actuarial disease free survival of 55%. The major causes of treatment failure have been GvHD and interstitial pneumonia with recurrent leukemia of lesser importance. This has led to a consideration of the possible antileukemic effect of GvHD or graft versus leukemia (GvHL). Experimental studies substantiate the GvHD effect in mice. However, reports of a decreased risk of leukemia relapse in patients with GvHD should be reviewed with reservation since there are no definite and reproducible criteria for defining GvHD (38,39). Moreover, the antileukemic effect of GvHD has not translated into a substantial survival advantage due to lack of an effective means of treating GvHD.

Clearly, marrow transplantation for AML in remission can substantially reduce the incidence of leukemic relapse. There is however, a substantial increase in early mortality associated with marrow transplantation. Preliminary analyses of controlled randomized trials comparing intensive chemotherapy to transplantation continue to indicate a decreased risk of leukemic relapse at two years in patients receiving transplants. Actuarial survival rates appear comparable by two years. The long term outcome of these trials is still uncertain and the role of bone marrow transplantation still remains controversial.

In summary, patients with AML are potential candidates for marrow transplantation during first remission. Although transplantation in remission reduces the risk of leukemic relapse it is still unclear whether survival is improved. Major problems remain to be addressed by prospective clinical trials in order to clearly define the role of transplantation in acute leukemia.

CHRONIC MYELOGENOUS LEUKEMIA (CML)

Survival of patients with CML has not changed substantially during the past two decades. Median survival is approximately 3 years and less than 20% of patients survive 5 years (40). Once the acute phase of the disease develops, therapy is generally unsuccessful and median survival is then less than 6 months (41). Some patients with CML may develop a transient "accelerated phase" characterized by fever, increasing basophilia and progressive hepatosplenomegaly. Survival from the onset of accelerated phase is only 3–6 months in most series (42).

Because of the overall poor prognosis of this disorder, bone marrow transplantation is being utilized as a therapeutic modality. Transplantation during the acute phase has been unsuccessful, generally because of inability to eradicate the leukemic cells or because of complications such as incomplete engraftment, GvHD, or interstitial pneumonia (43,44).

Recent reports of transplantation in chronic phase have been very encouraging. Eradication of leukemic clone with disappearance of the characteristic cytogenetic marker (Philadelphia chromosome) can be achieved with actuarial disease free survival rates of 70% at 3 years. Relapses have been rare (45–47) with actuarial continuous remission rates of 97%.

Results are much less satisfactory in patients transplanted in accelerated phase. Actuarial survival in this situation is 24% at 2 years (45).

In summary, the results of allogeneic marrow transplantation in CML appear very satisfactory in patients transplanted while in chronic phase. The procedure is associated with a substantial risk of severe complications which may be fatal. Because of these considerations, the optimal timing of transplantation is controversial. Prognostic factors can be determined in some cases (48) and these may be helpful in facilitating recommendation for transplantation in any individual patient.

REFERENCES

1. Bortin MM, Gale RP, Rimm AA. Bone Marrow Transplantation Registry. Allogeneic bone marrow transplantation in 144 patients with severe aplastic anemia. JAMA 1981;245:1132–9.
2. Gale RP. Clinical trials of bone marrow transplantation in leukemia. In: Gale RP, Fox CF, eds. The biology of bone marrow transplantation. New York Academic Press 1980:11–28.
3. Sparkes MC, Crist ML, Sparkes RS, Gale RP, Feig SA. Gene markers in human bone marrow transplantation. Vox Sang 1977;33:202–5.
4. Grebe SC, Streilein JW. Graft versus host reactions: A review. Adv Immunol 1976;22:119–221.
5. Von Bekkum DW. Immunologic basis of graft versus host disease. In: Gale RP, Fox DF, eds. The biology of bone marrow transplantation. New York Academic Press 1980:175–94.
6. Glucksberg H, Storb R, Fefer A, et al. Clinical graft versus host disease in human recipients of marrow from HLA-matched sibling donors. Transplantation 1974;18:285–304.
7. Slavin RE, Santos GW. The graft versus host reaction in man after bone marrow transplantation: Pathology, pathogenesis, clinical features and implication. Clin Immunol Immunopathol 1973;1:472–98.
8. Powles RL, Clink HM, Spence D. Cyclosporin A to prevent graft versus host disease in man after allogeneic bone marrow transplantation. Lancet 1980;i:327–9.
9. Weiden PL, Doney K, Storb R, et al. Antihuman thymocyte globulin (ATG) for prophylaxis and treatment of graft versus host disease in recipients of allogeneic marrow grafts. Transplant 1978;10:213–6.
10. Tutschka PJ, Beschorner WE, Hess AD, Santos GW. Cyclosporin A to prevent graft versus host disease: A pilot study in 22 patients receiving allogeneic marrow transplants. Blood 1983;61:318–25.
11. Granger S, Janossy G, Francis G, Blacklock H, Poulter LW, Hoffbrand AV. Elimination of T-lymphocytes from human bone marrow with monoclonal T antibodies and cytolytic complement. Brit J Haematol 1982;50:367–94.
12. Winston DJ, Bryson YJ, Ho WG, Territo MD, Golde DW, Gale RP. Interstitial pneumonia and cytomegalovirus infection after bone marrow transplantation. In: Gale RP, Fox CF, eds. Biology of bone marrow transplantation. New York Academic Press 1980:83–5.
13. Winston DJ, Ho WG, Champlin RE, Gale RP. Treatment and prevention of interstitial pneumonia associated with bone marrow transplantation. In: Gale RP, Fox CF, eds. Recent advances in bone marrow transplantation.

UCLA Symposia on Molecular and Cellular Biology, vol 7. New York: Alan R Liss Inc, Academic Press 1983:425–44.
14. Meyers JD, Flournoy N, Thomas ED. Nonbacterial pneumonia after allogeneic marrow transplantation: A review of ten years experience. Rev Infect Dis 1982;4:1119–32.
15. Kraemer KS, Neiman PE, Reeves WC, Thomas ED. Prophylactic adenine arabinoside following marrow transplantation. Transplant Proc 1978;141: 555–62.
16. Meyers JD, McGuffin RW, Neiman PE, Singer JW, Thomas ED. Toxicity and efficacy of human leukocyte interferon for treatment of cytomegalovirus pneumonia after marrow transplantation. Transplant Proc 1978;10:237–40.
17. Saral R, Burns WH, Laskin OL, Santos GW, Lietman PS. Acyclovir prophylaxis of herpes-simplex-virus infections: A randomized double blind controlled trial in bone marrow transplant recipients. N Engl J Med 1981;305:63–7.
18. Meyers JD, McGuffin RW, Bryson YJ, Cantell K, Thomas ED. Treatment of cytomegalovirus pneumonia after marrow transplant with combined vidarabine and human leukocyte interferon. J Infect Dis 1982;146:80–4.
19. Wade JC, Hintz M, McGuffin RW, Springmeyer SC, Connor JD, Meyers JD. Treatment of cytomegalovirus pneumonia with high dose acyclovir. Am J Med (suppl) 1982;73:249–56.
20. Winston DJ, Pollard RB, Ho WG, et al. Cytomegalovirus immune plasma in bone marrow transplant recipient. Ann Intern Med 1982;97:11–8.
21. Meyers JD, Leszczynski J, Zaia JA, et al. Prevention of cytomegalovirus infection by cytomegalovirus immune globulin after marrow transplantation. Ann Inter Med 1983;98:442–6.
22. O'Reilly RJ, Reich L, Gold J, et al. A randomized trial of intravenous hyperimmune globulin for the prevention of cytomegalovirus infections following marrow transplantation: Preliminary results. Transplant Proc 1983;15:1405–11.
23. Yeager AS, Grumet FC, Hafleigh EB, Arvin AM, Bradley JS, Prober CG. Prevention of transfusion acquired cytomegalovirus infections in newborn infants. J Pediatr 1981;98:281–7.
24. Camitta BM, Storb R, Thomas ED. Aplastic anemia: Pathogenesis, diagnosis, treatment and prognosis. N Engl J Med 1982;306:645–52.
25. Camitta BM, Thomas ED, Nathan DG, et al. A prospective study of androgens and bone marrow transplantation for treatment of severe aplastic anemia. Blood 1979;53:504–16.
26. Champlin RE, Ho WG, Winston DJ, Feig SA, Gale RP. Antithymocyte globulin treatment for aplastic anemia: A controlled randomized trial and comparison with marrow transplantation. Transplant Proc 1983;15:595–8.
27. Storb R, Doney KC, Thomas ED, et al. Marrow transplantation with or without donor buffy coat cells for 65 transfused aplastic anemia patients. Blood 1982;59:236–46.
28. Storb R (for the Seattle Marrow Transplant Team) Current status of marrow transplantation for the treatment of aplastic anemia. In: Gale RP, Fox CF, eds. Biology of bone marrow transplantation. New York: Academic Press 1980:1–10.
29. Storb R, Thomas ED, Buckner CD, et al. Marrow transplantation for treatment of severe aplastic anemia: Results in 20 "untransfused" patients. Ann Intern Med 1980;92:30–6.
30. Weiden PL, Storb R, Thomas ED, et al. Preceding transfusion and marrow graft rejection in dogs and man. Transplant Proc 1978;10:963–4.

31. Storg R, Hansen JA, Weiden PL, Clift RA, Thomas ED. Pretransplant lymphocytotoxins do not predict bone marrow graft rejection. Transplantation 1978;26:423–5.
32. Gluckman E. Pretransplant lymphocytotoxins and bone marrow graft rejection. Lancet 1978;i:443.
33. Ramsay NKC, Kim T, Nesbit ME, et al. Total lymphoid irradiation and cyclophosphamide as preparation for bone marrow transplantation in severe aplastic anemia. Blood 1980;55:344–6.
34. Parkman R, Rappeport J, Camitta B, Levey RH, Nathan DG. Successful use of multiagent immunosuppression in the bone marrow transplantation of sensitized patients. Blood 1978;52:1163–9.
35. Feig SA, Champlin RE, Arenson E, et al. Improved survival following bone marrow transplantation for aplastic anemia. Brit J Haematol 1983; 54:509–17.
36. Thomas ED, Sanders JE, Flournoy N, et al. Marrow transplantation in patients with acute lymphoblastic leukemia in remission. Blood 1979;56: 468–76.
37. Kanti RR, Holland JF, Glidewell OJ, et al. Treatment of acute myelocytic leukemia: A study by cancer and leukemia Group B. Blood 1981;58: 1203–12.
38. Weiden PL, Flournoy M, Thomas ED, et al. Antileukemic effect of graft versus host disease in human recipients of allogeneic marrow grafts. N Engl J Med 1979;300:1068–73.
39. McIntyre RM, Gale RP. Graft versus leukemia in man. In: Kunewick U, Meredith E, eds. Graft versus leukemia. Florida, CRC Press 1981:1–10.
40. Koeffler HP, Golde DW. Chronic myelogenous leukemia: New concepts. N Engl J Med 1981;304:1201–9 and 1269–74.
41. Cunningham I, Gee T, Dowling M, et al. Results of treatment of Ph+ chronic myelogenous leukemia with an intensive treatment regimen (L-5 protocol). Blood 1979;53:375–95.
42. Canellos GP. The treatment of chronic granulocytic leukemia. Clin Hematol 1977;6:113–28.
43. Fefer A, Cheever MA, Greenberg PD, et al. Treatment of chronic granulocytic leukemia with chemotehrapy and transplantation of marrow from identical twins. N Engl J Med 1982;306:63–8.
44. McGlave PB, Miller WJ, Hurd DD, Arthur DC, Kim T. Cytogenetic conversion following allogeneic bone marrow transplantation for advanced chronic myelogenous leukemia. Blood 1981;58:1050–2.
45. Champlin R, Ho WG, Winston DJ, Feig S, Gale RP. Allogeneic bone marrow transplantation for chronic myelogenous leukemia in chronic or accelerated phase. Transplant Proc 1983;15:1401–4.
46. Messner HA, Curtis JE, Nieman C. Allogeneic bone marrow transplantation in patients with CML prior to blast crisis. Blood (suppl) 1981;58:175A.
47. Doney KC, Buckner CD, Thomas ED, et al. Allogeneic bone marrow transplantation for chronic granulocytic leukemia. Exp Hematol 1981;9:966–71.
48. Tura S, Baccarni M, Corbelli G. Staging of chronic myeloid leukemia. Brit J Haematol 1981;47:105–19.

AUTOLOGOUS TRANSPLANATION OF BLOOD DERIVED HEMOPOIETIC STEM CELLS*

M. Körbling, Th.M. Fliedner

INTRODUCTION

The existence of circulating hemopoietic stem cells in the peripheral blood has been demonstrated by in vivo studies using preclinical animal models and by in vitro experiments. A bulk of data obtained in the canine model suggests that it would be possible to use stem cells collected from the peripheral blood of man for the purposes of hemopoietic reconstitution following an intensive cytoreductive pulse of pre-transplant therapy if adequate numbers of those cells could be harvested. The usual way of collecting a large amount of blood-derived hemopoietic stem cells is that of hemapheresis using a continuous flow blood cell separator.

There are both practical and theoretical advantages to the collection of stem cells from the peripheral blood over marrow harvest:

1. General anesthesia which is usually required for the collection of stem cells from the marrow space in man is not required for peripheral blood collections. This might be of importance in patients who are at poor riks for general anesthesia or whose marrow is damaged by previous radiotherapy.
2. The procedure of harvesting blood stem cells for transplantation purposes can be repeated several times without any harm to the donor.
3. Hemapheresis is a safe procedure, routinely done in blood banking.
4. Besides the advantage of easy stem cell procurement there is some evidence in myeloproliferative disorders that the ratio between normal hemopoietic stem cells and clonogenic tumor cells in favour of the first in the peripheral blood. If this turns out to be true, the use of blood stem cells would have a therapeutic advantage over marrow stem cells in the autologous transplant situation.

BLOOD STEM CELL PHYSIOLOGY

From the present evidence of hemopoietic development is seems, that the seeding of a bone marrow matrix by hemopoietic stem cells migrating via the blood stream is a principle that establishes itself during embryogenesis. This stem cell seeding can be repeated in adult life when a bone marrow with a normal cellular matrix and metabolic function becomes aplastic (1). From that it seems likely that the presence of stem cells in the peripheral blood is a physiologic necessity for the maintenance of an equilibrium among the stem cell pools in different marrow sites distributed throughout the

* Supported by the Tumor Center Heidelberg/Mannheim, West Germany.

sekeleton. If this concept is correct, then it appears logical to attempt the use of blood stem cells for therapeutic purposes.

PRECLINICAL CANINE MODEL

Animal models in the dog have been extensively developed and described by the Fliedner group. They have shown that infusions of cryopreserved blood-derived hemopoietic stem cells collected by use of the continuous-flow centrifuge, can avert the otherwise lethal effect of myeloablative therapy with total body irradiation (2). In several of these studies the number of granulocyte/macrophage progenitor cells (CFU-GM) was shown to correlate with the ability to reconstitute dogs from myeloablative therapy. It could further be shown that 80 to 90% of the mononuclear cells (MNC) and CFU-GM collected by means of hemapheresis did survive the cryopreservation procedure used for storage of these cells. In those preclinical transplantation studies hemopoietic progenitor cells have been stored successfully for periods in excess of 2 years and, at least in the canine model, such material has proved to be capable of restoring hemopoietic integrity.

To concentrate and purify blood-derived hemopoietic stem cells a technique was developed by the Fliedner group using different gradient centrifugation steps and providing a highly purified stem cell suspension. In a series of transplantation studies in the allogeneic situation, we could show, that after cryopreservation and thawing a volume of just 5 ml purified stem cell suspension was able to repopulate the complete hemopoietic system after myeloablative therapy. In those recipient dogs no signs of GvHD were seen which gives evidence to the fact that most GvHD inducing cells were separated out by the purification procedure (3).

COLLECTION OF PERIPHERAL BLOOD STEM CELLS IN MAN BY MEANS OF HEMAPHERESIS

In the clinical situation the collection of large quantities of blood stem cells in done by using a blood cell separator. In a series of 35 leukaphereses performed on adult volunteers 12×10^9 MNC and 8.7×10^5 CFU-C on the average could be harvested. The blood flow rate was adjusted to 50 ml per min and a total donor blood volume of 12 l was processed. The leukapheresis did not much affect the donor's blood cell concentration except the platelet

Table I. Yield of mononuclear cells (MNC) and hemopoietic progenitor cells per kg body weight harvested from marrow compared to peripheral blood.

		Marrow	Peripheral blood (n=12) (5 consecutive leukaphereses)
MNC	($\times 10^8$)	2–4	5.7–8.6
CFU-GM	($\times 10^4$)	5–20	4.3–6.2
BFU-E	($\times 10^4$)	4–35	-
CFU-GEMM	($\times 10^4$)	1–5	-

concentration which came down to around $100x10^9/l$. This decrease must be considered as a limiting factor for leukapheresis (4). While the concentration of CFU-C in the peripheral blood is only about one tenth that of bone marrow, it can be increased appreciably by previous chemotherapy and even by leukapheresis. Successive hemaphereses with short term intervals led to significant increases in CFU-C yield (4). The so far obtained total amount of leukapheresis derived MNC and CFU-GM is fairly comparable to the total cell yield harvested by multiple bone marrow aspiration (Table I). The i.v. administration of dextran-sulfate was shown to result in a fourfold to tenfold elevation of circulating CFU-C in the peripheral blood of dogs. Since the mononuclear cell count rose by a factor of two, a selective effect of dextran-sulfate on the circulating levels of committed myeloid precursor cells was suggested. Unfortunately a low molecular weight dextran-sulfate is not usable for clinical purposes because of its side effects (i.e. accumulation) (5).

CRYOPRESERVATION OF THE AUTOLOGOUS BLOOD STEM CELL GRAFT

The literature on autologous stem cell transplantation identifies many variables suggestive to have a significant effect on the overall efficiency of stem cell storage and recovery. Usually a controlled rate freezer is used which regulates the rate of cooling and prevents rewarming during the release of heat at the time of phase change. Dimethylsulfoxide is a widely used cryoprotectant which is added to the cell suspension to obtain a final concentration of 10%. The cell suspension is frozen at a cooling rate between 2 and 5°C per min in polyolefine-bags specially designed for ultralow temperature. To guarantee sterile handling under blood banking conditions we developed a plastic bag system for procurement, processing, freezing and thawing of the blood cell suspension (6).

A more critical question relates to the temperature at which stem cells are stored. In our experience a longer term decrease in stem cell viability (more than 5 months) can be averted if storage is carried out strictly at liquid phase temperature (-196°C) in liquid nitrogen. Although maximum storage times have not been established we know from marrow transplantation data that patients have received marrow cells stored up to 30 months with adequate hematologic reconstitution.

Storage of blood-derived mononuclear cells in liquid nitrogen using our cryopreservation technique allows a MNC and CFU-C recovery in the range of 90%.

There is still some controversy about how to thaw stem cells before reinfusion. Some use a stepwise dilution technique to mitigate the osmotic stress; others rapidly thaw the stem cells in a waterbath at a temperature between 37° and 50°C. The risk of clumping of thawed cell suspensions is increased by each DMSO-washing step and the time between thawing and reinfusion. To keep the risk at a minimum, some reinfuse the stem cell graft without washing out the cryoprotectant DMSO. Despite a temporarily unpleasant taste no major side effects have been observed sofar. The stem cell suspension is finally administered rapidly to the patient using a central venous line.

AUTOLOGOUS BLOOD STEM CELL TRANSPLANTATION

That hemopoietic engraftment can be achieved with human peripheral blood stem cells is well established. Goldman et al. first reported a clinical study using buffy coat autografts for patients with chronic myelogenous leukemia (CML) in transformation (7). We performed an autologous blood stem cell transplantation in a patient with chronic myelogenous leukemia with bone marrow cells containing the Philadelphia chromosome marker (Ph^1+) (8). After treatment with high dose cyclophosphamide, 26.3×10^9 blood mononuclear leukocytes, among them 26.2×10^5 granulocyte/macrophage progenitor cells (CFU-GM) were harvested by means of 5 successive leukaphereses when the bone marrow cells had been converted to Ph^1 negative. When the patient entered the aggressive phase (blast crisis), myeloablative treatment with busulfan (16 mg/kg) and cyclophosphamide (200 mg/kg) was given, followed by the transfusion of the cryopreserved blood leukocytes. Restoration of marrow and blood cellularity was completed about 20 days after this autologous blood stem cell transplantation. Marrow CFU-GM recovery was complete 2 weeks after transplantation, and all karyotypes of the patient's marrow cells were free of the marker chromosome.

CONCLUSIONS

The development of techniques for blood stem cell collection, processing, freezing, storage and thawing enables us to use blood derived stem cells as an alternative source for autotransplantation purposes. Such blood derived stem cell grafts can be given in addition to the marrow graft to augment the hemopoietic reconstitutive potency after myeloablative therapy and autologous bone marrow transplantation, especially to shorten the time of marrow aplasia and therefore to decrease the risk of septicemia. The blood stem cell graft can also replace the marrow graft in cases of damage to the marrow collection site. Finally blood stem cells can be collected and stored under preventive conditions from persons who are at risk for developing leukemia or for exposure to radiaton.

In conclusion the blood stem cell graft can be considered as a blood component like red blood cells or platelets, to be collected and cryopreserved in blood banks using their routine facilities, and delivered to the transplanters whenever they need it.

REFERENCES

1. Fliedner TM. Advances in hemopoietic stem cell research: their significance for clinical hematology. XII Congress of the International Society of Hematology, Paris, July 1978.
2. Fliedner TM, Calvo W, Körbling M, Nothdurft W, Pflieger H, Ross W. Collection, storage and transfusion of blood stem cells for the treatment of hemopoietic failure. Blood Cells 1979;5:313–28.
3. Körbling M, Fliedner TM, Calvo W, et al. Albumin density gradient purification of canine hemopoietic blood stem cells (HBSC): Long-term allogeneic engraftment without GVH-reaction. Exp Hematol 1979;7:277–88.
4. Körbling M, Fliedner TM, Pflieger H. Collection of large quantities of granulocyte/macrophage progenitor cells (CFUc) in man by means of continuous-flow leukapheresis. Scand J Haematol 1980;24:22–8.

5. Ross WM, Körbling M, Nothdurft W, Fliedner TM. The role of dextransulfate in increasing the CFU-C concentration in dog blood. Proc Soc Exp Biol Med 1978;157:301–5.
6. Körbling M, Fliedner TM, Rüber E, Pflieger H. Description of a closed plastic-bag system for the collection and cryopreservation of leukapheresis-derived blood mononuclear leukocytes and CFUc from human donors. Transfusion 1980;20:293–300.
7. Goldman JM, Catovsky D, Goolden AWG, Johnson SA, Galton DAG. Buffy coat autografts for patients with chronic granulocytic leukemia in transformation. Blut 1981;42:149–55.
8. Körbling M, Burke P, Braine H, Elfenbein G, Santos G, Kaizer H. Successful engraftment of blood derived normal hemopoietic stem cells in chronic myelogenous leukemia. Exp Hematol 1981;9:684–90.

THE ROLE OF AUTOLOGOUS BONE MARROW TRANSPLANTATION IN CANCER TREATMENT

G.L. Phillips

INTRODUCTION

Marrow transplantation is a method to reduce the hematological toxicity of ablative cytotoxic therapy; the immunologic problems of allogeneic marrow transplantation are avoided by using syngeneic marrow. Because identical twinning is rare, syngeneic marrow transplantation can be of chief benefit as an idealized model for autologous transplantation, a marrow source of ready availablity. The primary problem associated with syngeneic marrow transplantation for treating malignancy is not related to the marrow *per se*, but to the inability of the pretransplant ablative regimens to eradicate advanced cancer (1). Therefore the reinoculation of malignant cells in the autologous marrow, although worrisome, is of lesser immediate concern. Nevertheless, efforts to purge the marrow of tumor cells are important, and these efforts should parallel improvements in ablative regimens.

Additional problems of autologous marrow transplantation include delayed reconstitution of hematologic function in approximately 10 to 15% of cases, and the potential loss of an allogeneic reaction against the tumor cells. A syndrome resembling acute graft-versus-host disease with autologous marrow transplantation has been reported but is of uncertain significance. A problem common to all types of marrow transplantation for malignancy is the severe nonhematologic toxicity of the ablative treatment regimens.

Progress on these problems will allow full exploitation of autologous marrow transplantation as a major tool in the cytotoxic therapy of cancer.

RATIONALE UNDERLYING AUTOLOGOUS MARROW TRANSPLANTATION

The rationale underlying autologous marrow transplantation is listed in Table I and discussed below.

1. Increased doses of cytotoxic therapy have produced improved antitumor responses

This subject has recently been reviewed (2); evidence exists in experimental tumors, in human tumor systems in vitro, and to a lesser extent, in clinical trials that suggests a steep dose-response effect for most cytotoxic agents. This is especially true in tumors responsive to conventional-dose therapy. However, proof that marrow ablative doses of cytotoxic therapy alone produce superior results to conventional (if intensive) dose-therapy is scanty, and probably best represented by the syngeneic marrow transplant experience with refractory leukemia and lymphoma. In this situation,

Table I. Rationale underlying the use of autologous marrow transplantation for malignancy.

1. Increased doses of cytotoxic therapy have produced improved antitumor responses.
2. Hematological toxicity is dose-limiting for many antineoplastic agents; nonhematological toxicity is dose-limiting with marrow support.
3. Autologous marrow transplantation can reconstitute hematologic function after ablative therapy.
4. The disadvantages of allogeneic marrow transplantation are avoided.
5. The effects of reinoculating of small numbers of malignant cells are unknown.

even advanced disease is occasionally cured, a superior result compared to chemotherapy alone (3,4).

2. Hematologic toxicity is dose limiting for certain antineoplastic agents; nonhematologic toxicity is dose-limiting with marrow support

Tabel II is modified from Herzig's review (5). Various cytotoxic agents, their "usual dose", their "maximal dose without autologous marrow transplantation" and their "maximal dose with autologous marrow transplantation" are given. It also notes the dose-limiting nonhematologic toxicity of the

Table II. Dose escalation studies with intensive single-agent therapy and autologous marrow transplantation (AMT) (5).

Agent	Usual dose	Maximal dose without AMT	Maximal dose with AMT	Dose-limiting nonhematologic toxicity
TBI (rad)	150	350	1000 in 1 fraction or $<$ 1600 fractionated	Pulmonary
Cyclophosphamide (mg/kg)	50	200	200	Cardiac
BCNU (mg/m^2)	300	600	1200	Pulmonary, Hepatic
Mitomycin C (mg/m^2)	20	40	60	Hepatic
Nitrogen mustard	0.4	1.6	2.5	CNS
Melphalan (mg/m^2)	35	140	265*	Mucosal
AMSA (mg/m^2)	120	600	1000	Mucosal
VP16-213	500	1600	2400	Mucosal

* With cyclophosphamide "priming".

dose. Caution is required in interpretating this data; the usual dose (felt safe for outpatients) and the maximal dose without marrow transplantation (to the tolerance of hematologic supportive care) were in some cases determined before sophisticated supportive care was available. In these instances, doses in both categories could probably be increased somewhat, given the current ability to manage prolonged myelosuppression. Nevertheless, it is assumed that the myelosuppression produced by the maximal dose without marrow will not produce more than approximately 4 weeks of severe myelosuppression. The maximal dose with autologous marrow transplantation is limited by nonhematologic toxicity; a serious drug-related toxicity incidence of approximately 20% has been considered acceptable in treating an otherwise lethal malignancy (6), but this is admittedly arbitrary.

With this in mind, several features are observed:

a) Much of the "distance" between the usual and the maximal with marrow transplantation doses is in the area that does not require marrow support, i.e. between the usual dose and the maximal without marrow dose. For agents such as cyclophosphamide (7) no additional escalation is tolerated with marrow support, because of the appearance of dose-limiting nonhematologic toxicity. Even for agents in which a difference in dose exists between the two "maximal" doses (without and with marrow), it is often relatively small, i.e. twofold or less (e.g. BCNU, mitomycin C, nitrogen mustard, melphalan, AMSA, and VP16-213). Only for total body irradiation (TBI), where fractionated TBI doses of 1400 to 1500 rad can be given with marrow support is the difference afforded by marrow actually substantial (8). This suggests that a major benefit from single agent therapy is unlikely, regardless of dose, and new strategies using these augmented dose therapies are required before improved results can be regularly achieved. Options include combination chemotherapy with agents each used in ablative dose, and/or "adjuvant therapy" in the low tumor burden situation.

b) Dose-limiting nonhematologic toxicity is not always predictable from the experience with standard dose therapy; the cardiac toxicity noted with cyclophosphamide (7), and the hepatic toxicity of mitomycin C (9) illustrate this point. These toxicities are frequently fatal. With other agents, severe, yet nonfatal toxicity is dose-limiting; melphalan, approximately 225 mg/m^2 (10) and VP16-213, approximately 2400 mg/m^2 are examples (11), each producing severe mucosal toxicity.

c) The spectrum of nonhematologic toxicity observed with these agents at escalated doses is sufficiently broad to allow testing combinations. Many possibilities exist; we have combined melphalan (180 mg/m^2) plus BCNU (1200 mg/m^2) for treating malignant melanoma; preliminary data do not reveal increased toxicity compared to the intensive use of each agent alone (unpublished data). It is emphasized that the unpredictable toxicity noted with ablative-dose therapy requires an escalation phase preceding full-dose combination therapy. It is also desirable to evaluate new agents singly to avoid obscuring the presence of unanticipated toxic effects.

While antineoplastic agents frequently manifest their initial major toxicity as dose-related myelosuppression, marrow support is not required for all augmented dose-regimens. Hematologic recovery following successful syngeneic marrow grafting requires 2 to 4 weeks, and therapies that produce a shorter duration of marrow aplasia will not benefit from marrow support (7). Augmented dose therapy without marrow support can be used if eventual recovery of marrow function will occur; extensive supportive care is often capable of controlling pancytopenic complications for at least 4 weeks (12).

It is assumed, but not proven, that regimens including TBI doses of 1000 to 1575 rad, are fatal without marrow support (8) and little evidence exists to prove that any non-TBI containing regimen absolutely requires marrow support (5). However, the duration of myelosuppression may be shortened with nonmarrow-lethal regimens by using autologous marrow (12), and the intensive use of chemotherapeutic agents with profound toxicity to hematopoietic stem cells (e.g. carmustine, busulfan) may be marrow-lethal and marrow support is probably required (16). Marrow transplantation may also be indicated with regimens producing shorter intervals of pancytopenia if repeated use of the regimen (and cumulative myelotoxicity) is anticipated.

As noted in Table II, nonhematologic toxicity of the intensive use of these components often prohibits substantial escalation of dose even with marrow transplantation. Methods designed to reduce nonhematologic toxicity are being evaluated; fractionation of TBI is an example (13).

3. Autologous BMT can reconstitute hematologic function after ablative therapy

Unlike allogeneic transplants, the success of syngeneic and autologous marrow transplants cannot be proven by genetic markers. Therefore, the success of autologous marrow transplantation can be most convincingly demonstrated by hematologic recovery following marrow-lethal therapy; several studies have demonstrated that autologous marrow has this capability, even using marrow that has been exposed to cytotoxic agent therapy and cryopreserved for several years (5). Cryopreservation is important; storage of marrow in the liquid state beyond 4 or 5 days at most (14) is not possible, and in some instances, marrow storage for several years is desirable. Whereas optimal methods of cryopreservation are not known, the proper concentration of cryoprotectant and protein, controlled-rate freezing (with a short time spent at phase change), and storage at the lowest possible temperatures (15) are felt to be important.

Despite the absence of evidence that any regimen is marrow-lethal, successful recovery of marrow function following regiments that include TBI doses of 1000 rad or more is considered to be evidence of successful autotransplantation. This is even more convincing if the kinetics of recovery after autografting are parallel to those observed with normal marrow grafts

Table III. Comparison of engraftment of syngeneic versus autologous marrow transplantation following cyclophosphamide and TBI

Disease	Source	No.	Median day after transplantation PMN > 500/μl (range)	Platelets > 10-20,000/μl (range)
Acute leukemia (1)	Syngeneic	33	16 (11–29)	16 (10–58)
Malignant lymphoma (16)	Autologous	23	18 (12–37)	24 (10–67)

(5). (Likewise, marrow recovery that occurs beyond 4 to 6 weeks after autotransplantation cannot clearly be related to the marrow graft but may reflect endogenous recovery of residual marrow stem cells). Table III shows that the median day of marrow recovery was similar in 23 malignant lymphoma patients receiving cryopreserved autologous marrow (16) when compared to recovery in 33 acute leukemia patients (1) receiving fresh syngeneic marrow after similar cyclophosphamide and TBI therapy in both groups. This finding emphasizes that cryopreserved autologous marrow can reconstitute minimal hematologic function within 4 weeks of transplantation in most patients, even those with a history of previous chemotherapy or prolonged marrow storage (16). However, median recovery is delayed in occasional lymphoma patients and in many of our acute leukemia patients receiving identical ablative therapy and autologous marrow for an additional 10 to 14 days (5); possible mechanisms for this delay in marrow recovery include the effect of more intensive (antileukemic vs antilymphoma) therapies before storage or an intrinsic, persistent effect of leukemia in remission marrow. Although analysis of our data is incomplete, we believe that prior exposure to cytotoxic therapy is the primary problem, and marrow should be stored before extensive myelosuppressive therapy is administered.

4. The problems of allogeneic marrow transplantation can be avoided with autologous marrow

Superficially, it seems preferable always to use fresh, normal marrow for transplantation. The two major reasons why this is not possible are: 1) Most patients do not have suitable donors, and 2) the immunological problems of allogeneic marrow transplantation have a high morbidity and mortality (17).

Problems of the immunological rejection and GvHD are encountered even with using HLA-identical marrow, and many investigators have been reluctant to use less than HLA-identical marrow donors, reasoning that only inferior results would follow. However, recent studies using "mismatched" related or HLA-identical unrelated donors do not suggest an obvious increase in these complications (18). Even these additional marrow sources would not entirely eliminate the donor availability problem, however, and the unique complications noted with haploidentical transplants (19) suggest limits for "mismatched" marrow transplants.

Although graft rejection is uncommon in marrow transplantation for malignancy, potent immunosuppression is required in the allogeneic setting and the preparative regimen cannot be selected for its antineoplastic effects alone. Following engraftment, both acute and chronic GvHD occur frequently and are responsible for substantial morbidity and mortality (17). The presence of GvHD also leads to a variety of infections caused by delayed immunoreconstitution. Many of these problems are more severe in older patients, and the results of allogeneic marrow transplantation in patients older than 40 years of age are poor (20).

Many of these complications can be circumvented by the use of autologous marrow transplantation. Patients with a normal marrow status at virtually any point in their disease can undergo marrow cryopreservation, with the marrow kept in a viable state for at least several years until intensive therapy is required; therefore almost all patients can have "donors". Because graft rejection is not a consideration, agents may be selected on the basis of their cytotoxicity and side effects alone; improved antineoplastic results may be anticipated. Although acute GvHD has been reported with autologous marrow transplantation (20), the exact nature of this syndrome is uncertain and in any case rare; we have treated nearly 100 patients with cyclophosphamide, TBI, and autologous marrow transplants and only two have developed a clinical situation compatible with this diagnosis (unpublished data). Finally, avoiding GvHD may allow a reduction of the disabling infections, especially the cytomegalovirus-related interstitial pneumonitis that accounts for approximately 25% of mortality in some allogeneic series, but is less frequently seen in similarly treated patients receiving syngeneic (22) or autologous marrow transplants (16).

Autologous marrow transplantation is also associated with certain limitations; damage to marrow stem cells from therapy or the cryopreservation process can delay hematopoietic recovery, and inoculating occult tumor cells can prevent otherwise successful therapy. Each of these problems is reviewed elsewhere in this discussion. In addition, the loss of a beneficial graft-versus-tumor effect is possible (23).

5. <u>The effect of reinoculation of malignant cells in small number is uncertain</u>

This problem has been viewed as the major limitation of autologous marrow transplantation (17), and eventually, this is almost certain to be the case. However, that it is not the most immediate problem is emphasized by the observation that in only two circumstances (transplanting acute myelogenous leukemia in first remission or chronic myelogenous leukemia in stable phase) is the leukemic relapse rate less than 50% following intensive therapy and syngeneic marrow (1). The high failure rate of current regimens will obscure relapse caused by the reinoculated cells in the autologous marrow, and only recently has an adverse effect of occult leukemic cells in the transplanted marrow been demonstrated. Following intensive chemoradiotherapy, complete remission ($\approx$ 70%) and even median survival ($\approx$ 6 months) are similar in relapsed leukemia patients receiving either syngeneic or autologous marrow transplants. However, relapse occurred in 22/23 of the autografted leukemia patients by three years compared to 14/24 of the syngeneic marrow group, ($p < 0.01$, chi-square) (3, and unpublished data).

Therefore, occult leukemic cells in the autologous marrow contributes to a very high ($>$ 60%) relapse rate, and trials with more effective regimens will be required to demonstrate a favourable effect of dealing with the problem of marrow contamination (1). Two general approaches are possible. The first is avoidance, i.e. using of marrow in situations where it is unlikely to be contaminated, e.g. early in the course of a malignancy or in tumors that uncommonly spread to the marrow. A variation is to use more sensitive methods of detecting occult tumor in the marrow (24). Substantial problems are associated with this approach, including that the exclusion of malignancies most likely to have marrow contamination are those most responsible to current ablative regimens, i.e. the hematologic malignancies. Second, the presence of a "low" number of tumor cells in non-leukemic marrow is of unknown significance; at least three patients with marrow involved with lymphoma at diagnosis and later "converted" to remission status by conventional chemotherapy before storage have achieved prolonged disease-free survival (25).

A second approach involves removing malignant cells from the marrow, using physical, chemical, or immunologic methods (26). The main problem with this approach is the possibility of inadvertent damage to normal marrow

Table IV. Autologous marrow transplantation (AMT) for malignant lymphoma (26).

Series year(s)	NCI 1978	Paris 1981, 1983	Besancon 1983	Villejuif 1983	Seattle 1983	MD Anderson 1983	SECSG 1981, 1983
Number	22*	18	17****	16	11	6	53
Diagnosis							
Non-Hodgkin	22	16	17	14	7	4	40
Hodgkin	-	2	-	2	4	2	13
Disease status							
Remission	-	5	11	-	-	-	-
Relapse	22	13***	6	16	11	6	53
Regimen	BACT	BACT, TACC+ TBI	BACT, TACC	BACT	CY/ TBI*****	CBV (5) (CY/TBI (1)	CY/TBI (35) +LRT (18)
CR (%)	45	85	86	69	11	17	51
Toxic death (%)	18	6	24	19	81	34	23
DFS (%)	18**	39	42	31	-	17	21

* Includes 10 patients given BACT without AMT.
** Includes 2 patients with BM involvement at diagnosis.
*** Includes 3 patients treated at presentation.
**** Includes 1 patient given BACT without BMT.
***** Includes 3 patients who received modifications of CY/TBI.
****** Includes 1 patient with BM involvement at diagnosis.

Table V. Intensive nitrosourea chemotherapy and AMT for malignant glioma (26).

		No of glioma patients				
Series, year	Regimen mg/m²	Recurrent	Adjuvant	Responders %	No. alive, mos	Toxic death %
Hildebrand 1980	CCNU 390	7*	0	0	0	0
Carella 1981	BCNU 800	2	-	100	2(9+,7+,3+,3+)	0
		-	2	-		
Mortimer 1982	BCNU 1050–1200**	14**	-	56	1(24+)	21
Fingert 1983	BCNU 600–1400	18	-	28	4(41+,38+,32***,26+)	
Phillips 1983	BCNU 1050–1350	31	-	33	3(64+,31+,12+)	20
		-	7		3(45+,23+,4+)	0
Totals		72	9	-	13(64+–4+)	

* Includes two patients who did not receive AMT.
** Includes 12 patients who received concomitant 5-fluorouracil.
*** Recurrent diseases, currently free of disease following a second resection.

Table VI. Intensive therapy and ABMT for melanoma (26).

Institution	Remigen (mg/m^2)	No.	CR/PR	Survival (mos)	Toxic death
Royal	L-PAM (140)	20	2/9	6.5(4-11)	0
SECSG	BCNU (1200)	32	5/9	6.5(4-26+)	3
SECSG	L-PAM (180-225) (1400-1000)	15	5/5	7(3–12+)	2
University of Colorado	BCNU+L-PAM (35-110)(600-900)	18	2/6	11(2-34+)	1
SECSG	BCNU+L-PAM (90-180)	29	2/11	5(1-10+)	5
Totals		114	16/40		11

stem cells. Nevertheless, this approach is perhaps the most promising, especially with the ready availability, potential specificity, and wide spectrum of therapeutic possibilities connected with monoclonal antibody technology.

SUMMARY OF SELECTED CLINICAL TRIALS

1. Hematological malignancies

The curative potential of ablative therapy and syngeneic marrow transplantation in leukemia-lymphoma without the substantial mortality of allogeneic transplantation has stimulated interest in autologous marrow transplantation, as indicated in several recent reviews (1,5,25,27,28).

To illustrate the potential of autologous transplantation, results in the treatment of malignant lymphoma are outlined in Table IV. Patients were heterogeneous in histology, disease status, and treatment regimen, complicating a precise interpretation. However, a high complete remission rate and a 15 to 20% long-term survival of even resistant lymphoma patients was noted, confirming the syngeneic transplant experience (4). The treatment-related mortality is approximately 15 to 20%, the nonhematologic component of which is directly related to the ablative regimen; i.e. pulmonary with regimens containing TBI and cardiac with BACT or TACC (8).

Efforts to reduce toxicity and to improve antitumor efficacy have led to using syngeneic transplantation for leukemic patients in remission (29); however, the results of conventional treatment must justify the treatment-related mortality noted above, and it is generally agreed that few lymphoma patients in first remission are suitable candidates for this therapy (25). Patients other than those in advanced relapse or first remission are therefore optimal, i.e. have an overall poor prognosis but do not have the unfavourable features of far-advanced disease. Aggressive lymphoma in second complete remission, partial remission, and early relapse are examples of patients that should be promptly identified, evaluated, and considered for treatment with ablative therapy and autologous grafts.

In addition to earlier transplantation, the ablative regimens must be refined both to increase antitumor efficacy and to decrease toxicity. Examples include modifying (or even deleting) TBI to reduce toxicity, or adding local radiation or drugs; these efforts are being evaluated by various centres.

2. Solid tumors

Unlike the situation for the hematologic neoplasms, a standard therapy with curative potential (such as cyclophosphamide, TBI, and using syngeneic marrow) has not been convincingly demonstrated (1,25,28,30,31). Therefore, most solid tumor patients have received Phase I or early Phase II therapy (25,30). Nevertheless, some interesting results have been achieved in certain situations, e.g. using of high-dose BCNU (1000 to 1200 mg/m^2) in glioblastoma and melanoma (6,25, unpublished data) and high-dose melphalan (180-225 mg/m^2) in melanoma and neuroblastoma (10,32). Some of these results are illustrated in Table V and VI, demonstrating that long remissions are also possible in this group of refractory solid neoplasms.

SUMMARY

Syngeneic marrow transplantation is an idealized model for autologous marrow transplantation, a source of marrow that can be used with many more cancer patients than can syngeneic or allogeneic marrow; the donor unavailability problems of the former and the immunologic problems of the latter are avoided. Although reinoculating malignant cells with the autologous marrow is of concern, the primary problem underlying syngeneic marrow transplants for treating malignancy is the inadequacy (and to a lesser degree, the toxicity) of the ablative regimens. Efforts to refine these regimens must parallel those to rid the marrow of malignant cells for autologous marrow transplantation to reach its potential as a cancer treatment.

REFERENCES

1. Buckner CD, Stewart PS, Bensinger W, et al. Critical issues in autologous marrow transplantation for hematological malignancies. In: Gale RP, ed. Recent advances in bone marrow transplantation. New York: Alan R. Liss Inc, 1983:599–614.
2. Frei E, Canellos GP. Dose: A critical factor in cancer chemotherapy. Am J Med 1980;69:585–94.
3. Fefer A, Cheever MA, Thomas ED, et al. Bone marrow transplantation for refractory acute leukemia in 34 patients with identical twins. Blood 1981;57:421–30.
4. Appelbaum FR, Fefer A, Cheever MA, et al. Treatment of non-Hodgkin's lymphoma with marrow transplantation in identical twins. Blood 1981;58:509–13.
5. Herzig GP. Autologous marrow transplantation in cancer therapy. Prog Hematol 1981;12:1–23.
6. Phillips GL, Fay JW, Herzig GP, et al. Intensive BCNU and cryopreserved autologous marrow transplantation for refractory cancer: A Phase I–II study. Cancer 1983;52:1792–1802.

7. Buckner CD, Rudolph RH, Fefer A, et al. High-dose cyclophosphamide therapy for malignant disease. Cancer 1972;29:357–65.
8. Appelbaum FR, Thoma ED. Review of the use of marrow transplantation in the treatment of non-Hodgkins' lymphoma. J Clin Oncol 1983;1:440–7.
9. Lazarus HM, Gottfried MR, Herzig RH, et al. Veno-occlusive disease of the liver after high-dose mitomycin C therapy and autologous bone marrow transplantation. Cancer 1982;49:1789–95.
10. Lazarus HM, Herzig RG, Graham-Pole J, et al. Intensive melphalan chemotherapy and cryopreserved autologous bone marrow transplantation for the treatment of refractory cancer. J Clin Oncol 1983;1:359–67.
11. Wolff SN, Fer MF, McKay CM, et al. High-dose VP16-213 and autologous bone marrow transplantation for refractory malignancy: A Phase I study. J Clin Oncol 1983;1:701–6.
12. Appelbaum FR, Herzig GP, Graw RG, et al. Accelerated hemopoietic recovery following the infusion of cryopreserved autologous bone marrow in patients with lymphoma. Exp Hematol 1979;7(suppl 5):297–301.
13. Peters LJ, Withers HR, Condiss JH, et al. Radiobiological considerations in the use of total body irradiation for bone marrow transplantation. Radiol 1979;131:243–7.
14. Burnett AK, Tansey P, Hills L, et al. Hematological reconstitution following high-dose and supralethal chemo-radiotherapy using stored non-cryopreserved autologous bone marrow. Brit J Haemol 1983;54:309–16.
15. Buckner CD, Appelbaum FR, Thomas ED. Bone marrow and fetal liver. In: Karow AM, Pegg DE, eds. Organ preservation for transplantation. New York and Basel: Marcel Dekker Inc, 1981:355–426.
16. Phillips GL, Herzig RH, Lazarus HM, et al. Treatment of malignant lymphoma in relapse with cyclophosphamide, total body irradiation and cryopreserved autologous marrow transplantation. N Engl J Med 1984, in press.
17. Thomas ED. Marrow transplantation for malignant disease. J Clin Oncol 1983;1:517–31.
18. Hansen JA, Clift RA, Beatty PG, et al. Marrow transplantation from donors other than HLA genotypically identical siblings. In: Gale RP, ed. Recent advances in bone marrow transplantation. New York: Alan R Liss Inc, 1983:739–56.
19. Powles RL, Morgenstein GR, Crofts M, et al. Mismatched family bone marrow transplantation. In: Gale RP, ed. Recent advances in bone marrow transplantation. New York: Alan R Liss Inc, 1983:757–68.
20. Storb R, Prentice RL, Buckner CD, et al. Graft-versus-host disease and survival in patients with aplastic anemia treated by marrow grafts in HLA-identical siblings. N Engl J Med 1983;308:302–7.
21. Starke ID, Thein SL, Goldman JM, et al. Graft-versus-host disease after treatment for chronic granulocytic leukemic in transformation. Brit J Haematol 1982;52:383–7.
22. Appelbaum FR, Meyers JD, Fefer A, et al. Non-bacterial, non-fungal pneumonia following marrow transplantation in 100 identical twins. Transplantation 1982;33:265–8.
23. Weiden PL, Flournoy N, Sanders TE, et al. Antileukemic effect of graft-versus-host disease contributes to improved survival after allogeneic marrow transplantation. Transplant Proc 1981;13:248–51.
24. Benjamin D, Magrath IT, Douglas EC, Corash LM. Derivation of lymphoma cell lines from microscopically normal bone marrow in patients with undifferentiated lymphoma: Evidence of occult bone marrow involvement.

Blood 1983;61:1017–9.

25. Phillips GL. Current and clinical trials with intensive therapy and autologous bone marrow transplantation for lymphomas and solid tumors. In: Gale RP, ed. Recent advances in bone marrow transplantation. New York: Alan R Liss Inc, 1983:567–97.
26. Dicke KA. Purging of marrow cell suspensions. In: Gale RP, ed. Recent advances in bone marrow transplantation. New York: Alan R Liss Inc, 1983:679–88.
27. Zander AR, Dicke KA, Vellekoop L, et al. Autografting in acute leukemia. In: Gale RP, ed. Recent advances in bone marrow transplantation. New York: Alan R Liss Inc, 1983:689–702.
28. Herzig RH, Phillips GL, Lazarus HM, et al. Autologous bone marrow transplantation in the treatment of hematological malignancies. In: Wernick Ph, ed. Neoplastic diseases of the blood and blood forming organs. New York, Churchill Livingston, 1984 (in press).
29. Fefer A, Cheever MA, Greenberg PD, et al. Bone marrow transplantation (BMT) for acute leukemia with identical twins: Improved results with BMT in complete remission. Proc Asco 1983;19:182.
30. Kaye SB. Intensive chemotherapy for solid tumor — current clinical applications. Can Chemother Pharmacol 1982;9:123–33.
31. Spitzer G, Zander A, Tannir P, et al. Autologous bone marrow transplantation in human solid tumors. In: Gale RP, ed. Recent advances in bone marrow transplantation. Alan R Liss, Inc, New York 1983:615–42.
32. Herzig RH, Lazarus HM, Graham-Pole J, et al. Autologous bone marrow transplantation for malignant diseases: A Phase I–II study for melanoma, neuroblastoma, Ewing's sarcoma and germ cell tumors using high-dose melphalan. In: Gale RP, ed. Recent advances in bone marrow transplantation. New York: Alan R Liss Inc, 1983:643–57.

EVOLUTION OF SUPERIOR IMMUNE SUPPRESSION FOR HEART AND HEART-LUNG TRANSPLANTATION

B.P. Griffith, R.L. Hardesty, A. Trento, Ann Lee, H.T. Bahnson

INTRODUCTION

Conventional immune suppression protocols for heart transplantation were adapted from the successful use of azathioprine, prednisone, and antithymocyte globulin for kidney transplantation. Even in the leading centres, however, one-year survival rates following heart transplantation of only 60% were possible (1). Although lung and combined heart-lung transplantation appeared with the early flourish of heart transplantation in the late 1960s and early 70s, the lack of survivors delayed resurgence in these fields until superior immune suppression could be found (2,3). A superior form of immune suppression has been needed, and until the emergence of cyclosporine, improvements have not been possible (4).

Cyclosporine has been available since March of 1981 at the University of Pittsburgh as the major immune suppressant for 58 heart and 6 heart-lung transplant recipients. The initial 24 heart recipients received cyclosporine and low maintenance dose prednisone alone. This protocol was chosen as it had been responsible for excellent survival in our institution following liver and kidney transplantation (5,6). A specific avoidance of additional drugs such as azathioprine or antithymocyte globulin and the use of limited steroids was sought to minimize the potentially morbid side effects of over immunesuppression. Although the initial 6-month experience was encouraging (7), the 1 and 2 year survival rates fell to 61% and 41% respectively (8). Analysis of the causes of death indicated under immunesuppression, and thus antithymocyte globulin was added to the protocol in June 1982 as rescue therapy for recipients with severe or chronic moderate histologic rejection. This change has been a salutory one coincident with a 78% 15-month cumulative survival in the last 34 patients treated.

Heart-lung transplantation has been successful in all three patients treated for end-stage pulmonary vascular diseases but has failed in a similar number of patients with severe emphysema. These deaths have not been directly related to inadequate immunesuppression.

This manuscript is meant to identify the evolution of our current protocol for immunesuppression in patients receiving heart and combined heart and lung transplants. It is felt that the current results indicate the possibilities, limitations, and results of the transplantation of these organs.

PATIENT SELECTION

All 58 heart recipients were classified NYHA IV. All candidates were thought free from other systemic illnesses or recent pulmonary embolism. Two diabetic patients with low insulin dose requirements were transplanted, but generally diabetic patients were avoided. Recipient ages ranged between 6 and 55 years and averaged 39 years. Thirteen of these were female. Twenty-seven patients suffered from ischemic heart disease, 29 from idiopathic cardiomyopathy, and 2 from end-stage valve disease. Three patients with end-stage pulmonary vascular disease and 3 with severe emphysema underwent combined heart-lung transplantation. Two patients in the former group had primary pulmonary hypertension while the other suffered from Eisenmenger syndrome secondary to long-standing ventricular septal defect. One patient in the group with severe emphysema had α_1-antitrypsin deficiency.

ABO blood type was compatible in all cases. A lymphocyte crossmatch was desirable although a mismatch against donor lymphocyte (trypan blue) was recognized retrospectively in 5 patients. Interestingly, 2 of these mismatches occurred with a percentage of reactive antibodies of 0 (PRA 0%).

IMMUNESUPPRESSION

In the early experience, an oral loading dose of cyclosporine of 17.5 mg/kg was given just prior to transplantation, but oliguria soon after the operation, which did not seem related to the procedure, prompted a reduction in this loading dose to 10 mg/kg. Subsequent to transplantation the maximum dose tolerated was administered in 2 equally divided doses at 12-hour intervals, and that dose was limited by renal toxicity, less so by hepatic toxicity. The maintenance dose was usually adjusted so that the creatinine was 2 mg%, and rarely was a maximum dose of 17.5 mg/kg achieved (Table I). The blood

Table I. Immunesuppression cardiac TX 3/81–6/82.

Maintenance:
Prednisone 15–20 mg (10 d taper 200 mg)
Cyclosporine 5–10 mg/kg (max Cr $\leq$ = 2.5)
Rejection:
Hydrocortisone 1 gm

Table II. Immune suppression cardiac TX 7/83–present.

Maintenance:
Prednisone 15–20 mg (10 d taper 200 mg)
Cyclosporine 3–20 mg/kg
Whole blood RIA 700–1000
Rejection:
Mild/moderate – Medrol 1 gm
Severe/persistant – ATG

levels of cyclosporine were rarely used in the initial 24 patients, but in the last 16 months, whole blood levels of cyclosporine have been monitored by radioimmune assay (Sandoz), and oral doses have been adjusted to maintain trough levels between 800–1,000 ng/ml. The use of the blood levels has made the clinical management of patients easier, especially those with incipient renal failure and those requiring seizure control with phenobarbital or dilantin. Dose adjustments have become less empiric and more objective, and we believe this has improved clinical results by lessening toxicity. We are, however, unaware of any patient treated in the earlier experience with a creatinine of 2 in whom the initial blood levels were subtherapeutic.

Large initial doses of steroids were rapidly tapered to low maintenance levels. One gram of methylprednisolone was given as the circulation was restored to the heart recipient. In the heart recipients, prednisone, 200 mg/day in 2 divided doses, was started after the operation, and the daily dose was reduced by 20 mg each day to a maintenance dose of 20 mg daily by the 10th day. If oral medication was not possible, an equivalent dose of methylprednisolone was given intravenously (Table I).

Hydrocortisone, 1 gram intravenously, was used to treat rejection, usually without alteration of the dose of prednisone. The number and frequency of pulses varied depending upon the degree of rejection as determined by the endomyocardial biopsy. Severe rejection was treated with 3 daily doses of hydrocortisone, less severe with pulse doses at 3, 5, or 7 day intervals. Since July 1982, methylprednisolone has been substituted for hydrocortisone (Tables I, II).

While antithymocyte globulin was not used in the initial 24 patients, the immunesuppression regimen changed in July of 1982, and 34 patients were transplanted between then and October 1983. Moderate myocyte necrosis was initially treated with 3 daily pulses of methylprednisolone (1 gram), but if it did not resolve after 2 or 3 courses of this pulse therapy, 1 gram of rabbit antithymocyte globulin (Stanford) was administered daily for 3 days until the necrosis did resolve. Severe myocyte necrosis was immediately treated with a course of antithymocyte globulin (Table II). While T cells were monitored, their numbers and subset ratios were not used as an indication for the discontinuation of the empirically derived 3-day course.

Patients who received heart and lungs were treated with the usual cyclosporine doses, 125 mg of methylprednisolone every 8 hours for 1 day and 1.5 mg/kg/day of azathioprine for 21 days. Maintenance dose prednisone (20 mg) was substituted for the azathioprine after the initial 21 days. Mild rejection was treated with 1 or 2 intravenous pulses of methylprednisolone (1 gram), but those patients with endomyocardial biopsies suggesting persistent mild or moderate degrees of histologic rejection were treated with a 3-day course of antithymocyte globulin. The avoidance of steroids was desired in the favor of tracheal anastomotic healing.

OPERATIVE TECHNIQUE AND DONOR PROCUREMENT

Orthopic cardiac transplantation was performed utilizing a technique described by Lower and Shumway (9). Combined heart-lung transplantation was performed following example by Reitz et al. (10). The method of preservation of the donor heart prior to cardiac transplantation varied with respect to the use of cardioplegic solution. All grafts were immediately immersed and transported in a 4°C crystalloid solution. Most donor hearts were perfused with 1000 ml of crystalloid cardioplegic solution (4°C) before cardiectomy, and recently additional doses of blood cardioplegia have been given during implantation. The latter method has been associated with a reduced need for postoperative ionotropic support (11). Most hearts have been procured in conjunction with kidneys and/or livers. No adverse effects have been noted following multiple organ procurement. The techniques and results of multiple organ procurement have recently been described (12).

In all but 1 case, heart and lungs have been removed locally in an operating room adjoining that in which the implantation procedure has been performed. In 5 cases the donor has been core cooled on cardiopulmonary bypass and the posterior mediastinal dissection has been performed meticulously. Although a modified Collins solution (4°C) was used to flush the lungs, in the first three cases, our current preference is to rely upon in vivo cooling for lung preservation. We continue to use cardioplegic solution for myocardial preservation just prior to crossclamping the aorta.

RESULTS

The cumulative survival of the initial 24 patients at 1 year was 61% and at 2 years, 41%. Gratifyingly, however, since modification of the immunesuppression protocol to include rescue treatment with antithymocyte globulin since June 1982, a 78% 15 month cumulative survival has been achieved in 34 patients (Fig. 1). The initial series of 24 patients contained 4 deaths between 8 and 13 months due to chronic rejection and/or obliterative coronary artery disease, whereas 3 deaths resulted from acute rejection within the first 3 months. Only 1 patient treated since June 1982 has succumbed from rejection. This patient died suddenly and without antithymocyte globulin exposure on the sixth postoperative day prior to even the initial endomyocardial biopsy. The only clinical suspicion of incipient morbid

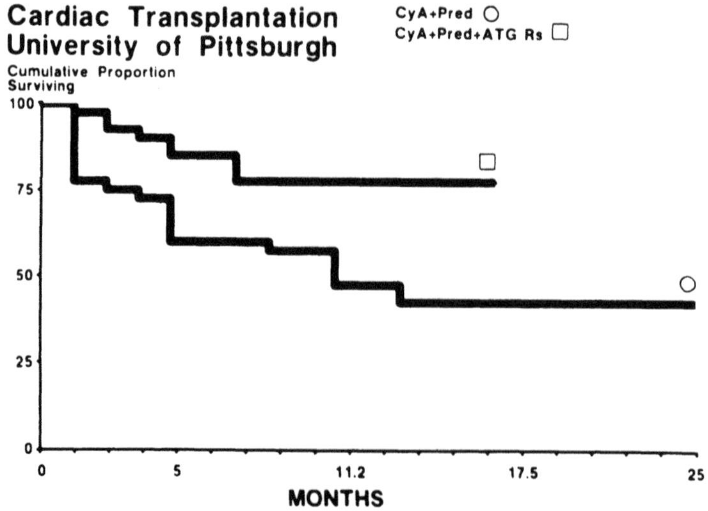

Figure 1.

rejection was a slight fall in the blood pressure 12 hours before sudden cardiac arrest.

Infection did not contribute significantly to mortality as only 2 patients in initial and 3 patients in subsequent group died with infection (Table III). Three patients in the initial group died from stroke within the first postoperative month. The first patient had sustained a cerebral embolism 10 days preoperatively from which he had nearly recovered. Postoperatively, there was an obvious extension of his cerebral injury. Another patient had been supported by balloon pump for 13 days preoperatively, and because of heparin allergy, could not be anticoagulated. At operation a blood clot was found extending from the left ventricle through the aortic annulus and beyond the aortic cross-clamp. Although initial recovery was apparent, 10 days postoperatively a sudden morbid cerebral embolism occurred. At autopsy, diffuse aortic thrombosis was noted. The last neurologically related death occurred in a 13 year old child 7 days postoperatively who succumbed from a diffuse intercerebral hemorrhage. Causative factors of this event remain unclear.

One heart recipient not exposed to antithymocyte globulin developed a diffuse cervical posterior pharyngeal lymphoproliferative disease and died with sepsis following treatment with multiple chemotherapeutic agents.

One patient treated since june 1982 died from rupture of an aortic dissection. It is believed that the origin of this dissection was at the cannulation site in the ascending aorta.

Two of 3 patients treated for pulmonary vascular diseases with combined heart-lung transplantation are well 6 and 14 months postoperatively. The other patient in this category died at 4 months subsequent to a small bowel perforation caused by an extensive lymphoproliferative disorder (Table IV). Prior to the development of this lymphoproliferative disorder, this patient

Table III. Cause of death of 18 patients (out of 58) receiving two therapy regimens.

Regimen: cyclosporine, prednisone (24 patients, 13 deaths)		Regimen: cyclosporine, prednisone, rescue ATG (34 patients, 5 deaths)	
Infection (2)	E. coli peritonitis (3 mo) E. coli pneumonia (9 days)	Infection (3)	Listeria meningitis (4 mo) Mixed lung abscess (2 mo) CMV pneumonitis and Aspergillus brain abscess* (6 mo)
Rejection			
(3 acute)	(1 o, 1½ mo, 2½ mo)		
(4 chronic)	4 x (12 mo)	Rejection (1)	(6 days)
Other		Other (1)	Aortic dissection (2 mo)
(3 stroke)	(7 days, 14 days, 1 mo)		
(1 lymphoma)	(11 mo)		

* Lymphoma nodules found in lungs and kidney at autopsy.

Table IV. Fate of 6 patients receiving heart-lung transplants.

Patient	Disease	Outcome
1	emphysema	died: 3D (inadequate lung preservation)
2	primary pulmonary HT	alive: 14 mos
3	emphysema	died: 1 mo (disseminated candidiasis)
4	primary pulmonary HT	died: 4 mos (lymphoproliferative disease)
5	emphysema	died: 3 mos (seizure)
6	Eisenmenger VSD	alive: 6 mos

had returned home and was leading a normal existence. All 3 patients with emphysema died within 3 months. The first was lost from inadequate ex-vivo lung preservation following an ill-advised attempt at distant heart-lung procurement. Another died from thoracic, mediastinal, and metastatic candidiasis contracted from a prolonged bronchopleural fistula. The last patient succumbed from a persistent seizure abnormality 10 weeks postoperatively. This patient, however, convincingly demonstrated an ability to maintain a normal pattern of ventilation in spite of the significant thoracic and diaphragmatic architectural derrangement common to patients with end-stage emphysema. No cause for the persistent seizure activity was identified.

REJECTION

Histologic rejection was monitored by endomyocardial biopsies obtained weekly during the first 6 weeks postoperatively and thereafter on an out-patient basis usually once a month during the first 6 months. Electrocardiographic voltages, arrthymias, clinical criteria of low cardiac output, cardiac sounds, and T-cell subsets were not useful in the detection of early rejection.

The most important aspect of the initial experience in the 24 patients was that persistent histologic rejection with focal myocyte necrosis was not reversed with pulse therapy of steroids (hydrocortisone) or with an increased dose of maintenance prednisone (30–40 mg/day). Consequently, 3 patients died with acute rejection within 3 months and 4 additional patients with chronic rejection and restrictive cardiomyopathy within 14 months. The rejection deaths prompted the addition of antithymocyte globulin if myocyte necrosis could not be eliminated by pulse of steroid. Fifteen of the 34 patients operated upon since June 1982 have received at least one 3-day course of antithymocyte globulin. Four patients required 2 courses, 3 patients 3 courses and 1 patient 4 courses before reversal of rejection. In spite of the earlier moderate to severe acute and/or chronic histologic rejection, none of these patients currently have evidence of persistent rejection or impaired graft function, and thus this group is distinctly different from those who received repeated pulses of steroids alone in response to severe and chronic moderate rejection. Rejection has been infrequent and mild beyond 6 weeks postoperatively. Both the initial and the latter groups have averaged 6 pulses of intravenous steroids for the treatment of rejection during the initial hospitalization. The 7 patients in the initial series with severe or chronic moderate rejection succumbed after averaging 13 steroid pulses.

Combined heart and lung recipients have demonstrated only mild histologic myocardial rejection. Although 3 of these patients have received antithymocyte globuline, they have so on the belief that T-cell modulation is less detrimental to tracheal healing than the early administration of pulse steroids. Radiographic evidence of lung rejection has not occurred in the absence of myocardial histologic rejection.

Mismatch against donor lymphocytes was known after implantation of the donor heart in 4 of the initial 24 and in 1 of the last 34 patients. No patient died of hyperacute rejection, and 3 of the 4 not treated with antithymocyte globulin survived and are free of chronic rejection. Two patients died of rejection, however, within 2 months.

INFECTION

Infection was studied in 35 consecutive patients (13), and although 9 patients' deaths were associated with infection, only 4 were specifically attributed to the infection. Some of these fatal infections occurred in the context of other morbid transplant problems including rejection, CMV pneumonitis, and lymphoma. Seventy-six per cent of the patients had at least one symptomatic infection, and there were a total of 52 infections in this group, 1.5 per patient. Within the first 3 months, the frequency of infection episodes was 0.8, with a steady drop to 0.1 per quarter 1 year post transplantation. Bacteremia occurred in 8 patients (6 deaths) for a total of 10 episodes; 7 were caused by Gram-negative rods and 3 by Gram-positive bacteria. Although the incidence of infection correlated with severe rejection, it did not appear to be related to patient age or the diagnosis of pretransplant heart disease. Patients with severe rejection had a mean of 2.33 infection episodes per patient while 21 with more moderate rejection experienced 1.14 episodes per patient ($p < 0.01$). Since rescue ATG was incorporated into our immune suppression protocol, patients with severe rejection have received less steroid pulse therapy, and their infection rates have been lower. Interestingly, there have been no deaths attributable to infection among those treated with ATG. Herpes viruses and bacteria account for almost 90% of all pathogens identified in symptomatic infections, and there has been a surprisingly low incidence of fungal infection. One patient was cured of mediastinitis caused by Staph. epidermidis and Candida albicans while another died of CMV pneumonitis and Aspergillus brain abscess.

HYPERTENSION

It has been noted in our series that hypertension has occurred in nearly all surviving patients who received cyclosporine in spite of all known pretransplant risk factors (14). The hypertension has been associated with normal cardiac output and abnormally elevated systemic vascular resistance, a distortion of neurogenic control, and a modest impairment of renal function leading to an increase in intravascular volume due to an impairment in sodium excretory function. Renin and urinary catecholamine levels have been normal. The approach to treatment has been systematic incorporating the use of diuretics to reduce intravascular volume, vasodilators to reduce vascular tone and sympatholytic drugs to attenuate the effects of circulating catecholamines. Recently, the calcium channel blocking agent, niphedipine, has been tried with some success. No current regimen appears to be totally satisfactory although some improvement has been noted.

RENAL TOXICITY

Renal insufficiency has often occurred postoperatively. Since the measurement of cyclosporine whole blood levels by radioimmune assay, the incidence of early postoperative oliguria has been decreased, but most of all patients show evidence of an elevated BUN and creatinine upon discharge from their initial hospitalization. The average maximum postoperative serum creatinine was 3.5 mg/100 ml with a corresponding BUN of 75 mg/100 ml. At discharge these values averaged 1.4 and 35 respectively. As out patients, patients were noted to have an increasing renal impairment as their serum creatinines averaged 2.2 mg/100 ml at 6 months. This trend has continued in spite of dose reductions in cyclosporine to reach 500–800 ng/ml.

LYMPHOPROLIFERATIVE DISEASE

Three of 58 heart recipients and 2 of 6 heart-lung recipients have developed a lymphoproliferative disorder indistinguishable from a mixed histiocytic lymphocytic lymphoma. These disorders have been noted within the first 4 months postoperatively in all cases. Three and perhaps 4 of these 5 have contained Epstein-Barr nuclear antigen (EBNA), suggesting an association with Epstein-Barr virus infection. A heart-lung transplant recipient died with a diffuse lymphoproliferative disorder without evidence of EBNA. Clonal status has been difficult to interpret, and its meaningfulness has been questioned as 2 patients have been monoclonal and 2 patients have been polyclonal. The remaining patient's status has not been determined to date.

One heart recipient and 1 heart-lung recipient have succumbed from the disease. The heart recipient was treated with multiple chemotherapeutic agents and died with sepsis and pancytopenia. Subsequent to that patient's course, we have adopted the attitude that the disorder is a disease of over-immunesuppression, and that the treatment should be primarily one of lowering the immunesuppression. Currently, patients who demonstrate evidence of this lymphoproliferative disorder are placed on 1–2 mg/kg/day of cyclosporine and low prednisone doses. They are followed very closely for the appearance of rejection. Using this treatment protocol, we have noted regression and apparent cure of tumor in 2 patients. The heart-lung recipient who died did so as a consequence of a small bowel perforation, but there was a striking decrease in the amount of tumor noted at autopsy as compared to that diagnosed prior to the reduction in his immunosuppression.

The fifth patient succumbed from CMV pneumonitis, and his EBNA staining tumor was unexpected at autopsy and found throughout his lungs.

At the present time the importance of Epstein-Barr viral surveillance is uncertain, but in the presence of serologic conversion or reactivation in favor of Epstein-Barr viral infection, patients are treated with the acyclic curing antimetabolite, acyclovir. The impact of this treatment is unknown at the present time. Current studies are focusing upon the effect of cyclosporine upon gastrointestinal proliferation in the rat. It may be that cyclosporin A induces extensive B-cell proliferation in response to many different types of infections and that this proliferation is responsible for the clinical entity now termed lymphoproliferative disorder. It would appear that at the present time an appropriate clinical step in the management of patients who develop this disorder should include reduction of immunesuppression with the avoidance of multiple chemotherapeutic antimetabolite agents.

CONCLUSION

Clearly, we have noted the evolution of an improved protocol for immunesuppression following heart and heart-lung transplantation. Through the use of cyclosporine, low-dose prednisone, and rescue antithymocyte globulin, one might anticipate survival rates approaching 80% following cardiac transplantation. Heart-lung transplantation now appears to be a clinical reality as cyclosporine seems to have provided an essential improvement and permits the avoidance of steroid medication within the critical first 3 weeks postoperatively. It is common dictum that multiple drug therapy should be avoided if possible so that over-immunesuppression and all of its attendant complications can be avoided. Because in the initial group treated with cyclosporine and prednisone alone, 30% succumbed from the effects of severe rejection. It was obvious that an additional agent would be necessary. Antithymocyte globulin has ably filled that requirement, and nearly 50% of the last 34 patients have required rescue treatment with this additional agent. We contend that prophylactic use of antithymocyte globulin is not necessary and that between 30 and 50% of patients treated might ultimately require it if long-term survival is to be anticipated.

With the evolution of this new immunosuppression protocol, we have noted the appearance of a yet to be understood diffuse lymphoproliferative disorder indistinguishable histologically from a mixed histiocytic lymphocytic lymphoma, a poorly understood tendency for hypertension, and almost universal mild renal toxicity. Bacterial and viral infections continue to occur although morbid infections have not been prevalent. Fungal infections have not occurred as commonly as in those patients receiving conventional immunesuppression with azathioprine and prednisone therapy.

Heart-lung transplantation is certainly emerging as a very therapeutic operation for patients with pulmonary vascular disease, and it would be anticipated that 80% survival rate should be achieved in those centres experienced with this operation and following similar immunesuppression protocols. Expansion of the selection criteria for heart-lung transplantation to include patients with parenchymal diseases has not provided long-term survivors even though one patient in this series has demonstrated a convincing ability for normal ventilation in spite of severe thoracic and diaphragmatic distortion.

Further improvements in immunesuppression have yet to emerge for clinical use, yet the expansion of monoclonal antibodies may provide an opportunity for selective immunesuppression. Such a "silver bullet" might make organ transplantation universal as the deleterious side effects of more global immunesuppression might be avoided.

REFERENCES

1. Baumgartner WA, Reitz BA, Oyer PE, Stinson EB, Shumway NE. Cardiac homotransplantation. Curr Probl Surg 1979;16:1–61.
2. Veith FJ. Lung transplantation. Surg Clin North Am 1978;58:357–64.
3. Cooley DA, Bloodwell RD, Hallman GL, Nora JJ, Harrison GM, Leachman RD. Organ transplantation for advanced cardiopulmonary disease. Ann Thorac Surg 1969;8:30–42.
4. Borel JF, Feurer C, Magnée C, Stähelin H. Effects of the new antilymphocytic peptide cyclosporin A in animals. Immunology 1977;32:1017–25.
5. Starzl TE, Weil R III, Iwatsuki S, et al. The use of cyclosporin A and prednisone in cadaver kidney transplantation. Surg Gynae Obs 1980; 151:17–26.
6. Starzl TE, Klintmalm GBG, Porter KA, et al. Liver transplantation with the use of cyclosporin A and prednisone. N Engl J Med 1981;305:266–9.
7. Griffith BP, Hardesty RL, Deeb GM, Starzl TE, Bahnson HT. Cardiac transplantation with cyclosporin A and prednisone. Ann Surg 1982;196:324–9.
8. Griffith BP, Hardesty RL, Bahnson HT. Powerful but limited immune suppression for cardiac transplantation with cyclosporin and low dose steroid. JTCUS 1984;87:1:35–42.
9. Lower RR, Shumway NE. Studies on orthotopic transplantation of the canine heart. Surg Forum 1960;11:18.
10. Reitz BA, Pennock JL, Shumway NE. Simplified operative method for heart and lung transplantation. J Surg Res 1981;3:1–5.
11. Hardesty RL, Griffith BP, Deeb GM, Bahnson HT, Starzl TE. Improved cardiac function using cardioplegia during procurement and transplantation. Transplant Proc 1983;15:1253–5.
12. Shaw BW, Rosenthal JT, Griffith BP, et al. Techniques for combined procurement of hearts and kidneys with satisfactory early function of renal allografts. Surg Gynae Obs 1983;157:261–4.
13. Dummer JS, Bahnson HT, Griffith BP, Hardesty RL, Thompson ME, Ho M. Infections in patients on cyclosporine and prednisone following cardiac transplantation. Transplant Proc 1983;15:2779–81.
14. Thompson ME, Shapiro AP, Johnson M, et al. New onset of hypertension following cardiac transplantation: A preliminary report and analysis. Am J of Cardiol 1983;51:489–91.

DISCUSSION

Moderators: G. Opelz, D. v.d. Waaij

G. Opelz:

Dr. Wood, could you compare the effect on kidney rejection of cyclosporin A to conventional therapy? What is the state of the art there?

R. Wood (Oxford, United Kingdom):

According to the mechanism of action of cyclosporin A, you would think that there should not be a role for the drug in treating acute rejection. However, various units have used cyclosporin A in this way, particularly the group in Halifax (McDonald et al. 1983)*, and they have shown quite good results. There may be a group of patients in whom the rejection process is not being adequately controlled by azathioprine and prednisolone and reversal can be achieved by the introduction of cyclosporin A. The problem is to identify which patients will benefit when cyclosporin A is used in this way.

G. Opelz:

Dr. Krom, if I understood correctly, you are somewhat sceptical about the improvement of results that has been attributed to cyclosporin A. In the improved survival curves of the Pittsburgh Group, have those patients been repeatedly transplanted? As you have noted, there was a large fraction of retransplanted patients. Are these included in the survival curve as successes, or is that a curve for first grafts only?

It makes a difference whether you can make a graft work for a long period of time by administering cyclosporin A, or whether you lose it every three months and have to retransplant a new liver.

R.A.F. Krom:

In liver transplantation we are not talking about graft survival or patient survival separately, because most of the time it is completely related.

G. Opelz:

That makes it somewhat less impressive, if you have to transplant someone three times to get a six months survival statistic.

* McDonald AS, Beletsky P, Cohen A, et al. Cyclosporine for steroid-resistant rejection in azathioprine-treated renal graft recipients. Transplant Proc 1983;15:2535–7.

R.A.F. Krom:

There is one good thing in Pittsburgh: They have so many donors available that they do not want to treat patients endlessly for just supporting life in a liver rejection. As soon as the patient is not really doing well, they are more eager to retransplant. Therefore, you will never know what could happen if the patient was treated regularly for rejection.

B.P. Griffith (Pittsburgh, U.S.A.):

It is my understanding that a number of the retransplants were performed before cyclosporin A levels where being routinely obtained in Pittsburgh. As you know cyclosporin A absorption is critically related to gastro-hepatic function. In part, the retransplantation rate may fall as more intravenous cyclosporin A is given. So far, it was always given by mouth.

A.B. Glassman:

Dr. Griffith, could you comment on the incidence of lymphoproliferative disorders? This is one of the side-effects of which not much was said about by any of the speakers. As I remember Pirosky and Dansen* described lymphoproliferative disorders, including lymphosarcomas in some transplant patients who had been given antilymphocyte globulin. Do you think this was related to the addition of ATG, or have you seen it previously?

B.P. Griffith:

It is related to overimmunosuppression, by whatever way you define that. It may not be necessary to define over-immunosuppression by the addition of a third agent. We have had half of our lymphoproliferative disorders show up in cardiac patients not exposed to ATG, but exposed only to low-dose steroids and cyclosporin A. Of our six cases, three have had no staining for Epstein-Barr. Perhaps a fifth, clearly a sixth was not positive for Epstein-Barr virus. They have occurred in our group within four months. We treated one patient with multiple chemotherapeutic agents, with a result of a pancytopenia and a death from sepsis. Subsequent to that experience, all patients have been treated as if they had been over-immunosuppressed. Two cases have had clear improvements with that type of homeopathic doses of cyclosporin A, and are well without evidence of tumor. Another patient had clearly resolved a large bulk of tumor just with the reduction in immunosuppression, but perforated a small bowel and died from that.

Speaking with collaborators at Stanford, in the heart group, because that is where my experience is, there appeared to be a correlation with cyclosporin A level and intensity of T-cell depletion, in those patients who had T-cell depletion over a length of time. Those patients who got them and formed them in the early Stanford experience, and all those treated at Stanford with cyclosporin A also got prophylactic ATG for three courses. That group came down with almost a 20% incidence of lymphoma. In that group, the patients who got the lymphoma were those patients who had the highest cyclosporin A levels and the lowest T-cell numbers for the longest time. So, clearly it is related. Whether it is a uniform infection or only Epstein-Barr, I do not know.

* Postgrad Med J 1976;52 (suppl 5):51–4.

W.G. Ho:

On the same subject, our experience with ATG in patients with aplastic anemia extends over about 80 patients who have been treated with this immunosuppressive agent. We have not seen any lymphoproliferative disorders, but the difference may still be that because the course of ATG that is given is not very prolonged.

I would like to ask a question to anyone, who also uses ATG for one reason or another. We see in practically every patient who receives ATG for aplastic anemia some form of serum sickness. I wonder whether this is observed in the renal transplant, the kidney transplant, or any of the other organ transplants.

B.P. Griffith:

What kind of ATG are you using?

W.G. Ho:

We are using a preparation from the Upjohn Company. This is an anti-thymocyte globulin that is produced by immunizing horses with human thymocyte or T-cells. The globulin factor is separated and partially purified and this is what is used as anti-thymocyte globulin (ATG).

B.P. Griffith:

We have not seen it.

G.F.J. Hendriks:

Many interesting data about heart, liver, and kidney transplantation were presented during this symposium. One of the fascinating differences between these groups is the incidence of early graft rejection. As Dr. Krom showed, this incidence of graft rejection in the groups of patients receiving a liver transplant is 10%. From experiments in the rat model it was shown that this low incidence of liver graft rejection is due to the fact that the autologous liver had been removed at the time of transplantation. Looking at the human data, presented by Dr. Krom, it also appears that by removing the autologous liver, the recipients immune response against allogeneic liver graft determinants seems to be less strong.

R. Wood:

I think that may be true but rates of graft survival may also be affected by the extent of Class II antigen expression on the cells of different organs and variation in the numbers of dendritic cells they contain. For example, there is a high level of expression of Class II antigens on renal tubules, while the hepatocytes of the liver and the myocardial cells of the heart are negative. This might partly explain why the kidney appears to be more readily rejected than the heart or liver.

B.P. Griffith:

One other thing that has to be mentioned is a hard-learned lesson in Pittsburgh. If you lose half of your heart function, you really have a functionless organ. So, the amount of rejection required to diagnose a rejection episode clinically and the amount of rejection which ends in the loss of your patient perhaps is less than that which a liver can sustain. The regenerative power of the liver does not exist for the heart. A lost muscle is a lost muscle and is replaced by fibrous tissue. I think this is why the heart group will see more lymphoproliferate disease, more complications from overimmunosuppression.

G. Opelz:

Dr. Krom, you mentioned that the Pittsburgh Group, with so many livers available, could do a lot of liver transplants. Are you implying that there are not many livers or not enough livers here, and what are the reasons for this? What are the problems?

R.A.F. Krom:

I do believe we have enough donors here, but people do not realize that there is a larger demand for organs than just kidneys. It has been done in the larger centres, but in the smaller donor hospitals the problem of getting organs other than kidneys still exists.

G. Opelz:

I would like to ask both Dr. Krom and Dr. Griffith: Do you have a waiting list and how big is it?

R.A.F. Krom:

We are a starting centre and our waiting list for patients who are ready for transplantation is 6 at the moment.

B.P. Griffith:

The heart-lung programme has a waiting list which is in the neighbourhood of 20, simply because of the unavailability of donors. We suspect that we can only do about 5 a year, because of the problem of local donations. The heart program has less of a list, fluctuating between 3 and 10 perhaps.

C.H. Gips:

Dr. Griffith, in the long-term survivors in the liver transplantations, we are at a median of 20 mg of prednisolone after one year, at 15 after two years, and 10 after four years. How is this in the cardiac transplants? Who gets cyclosporin A and prednisolone?

B.P. Griffith:

Our experience has been similar in terms of a taper. At about 6 months the patients are tapered from 20 mg to 15. We have seen very little complications from daily doses of 15 mg steroid. We have just been a little bit worried about losing good results.

C.H. Gips:

Could you imagine that, after one or two years, you could use azathioprine as well in low doses, or do you think that you need cyclosporin A plus prednisone in the proportions that we use with azathioprine?

B.P. Griffith:

I just do not know, but my impression is that we could get away with using less steroid after a year.

J.P. Hester:

Dr. Ho, and perhaps Dr. Phillips, what are your current recommendations on transplanting CML in the benign phase with allogeneic donors? Do you have a prognostic factor to find that level?

W.G. Ho:

I was expecting this question. Since we feel that the results of transplantation for CGL in the chronic phase are very good, our current policy is to explain to patients at the time of diagnosis that if an HLA-identical donor is available, bone-marrow transplantation is not an unreasonable way of approaching the treatment from that time. The actual decision, however, is made at a conference meeting with the patient and everyone concerned. So, we feel that it is not unreasonable to propose bone-marrow transplantation even from the time of diagnosis, until further data are related to the prognosis of the full group of patients.

C.L. Phillips (St. Louis, U.S.A.):

We transplant patients in stable condition, provided it has been one year from their diagnosis.

C.Th. Smit Sibinga:

I would like to make a few more comments. First of all, there was one particular subject on which we have not touched deliberately. All the organs being discussed here in transplantation, starting with the blood, going to the bone-marrow, the solid organs – particularly the kidney and the liver – finally ending with the heart and lungs, deal with donors who are willing to share, or to donate them depending on the kind of organ. As this is so, one could state that basically, these organs form a kind of national or even international resource. They are available in abundant quantities. The question is: How do we get access to them and how are we going to find the willingness to share them or to offer them? Basically, all these organs are being given on a voluntary and non-renumerated basis, although the voluntarism is morally biased, particularly when we deal with relatives of the patients. Secondly, all these organs have to meet specific criteria as to their procurement, preservation and ultimately their transplantation. What we have not touched is the aspect of morality and the legal aspects in protecting both donors and patients. The importance is in the fact that there are already brokers on the market who are trying to "catch" organs for selling them worldwide. This is a development which is very unfortunate. We should be well aware of this.

G. Opelz:

We have had two very interesting days. They were informative, they were productive. I have learned a lot and I do hope that all of you have learned something during these two days.

I would like to thank all of you, for having been an active, interested and responsive auditorium in the discussions. I have enjoyed these two days very much, and I would like to thank Dr. Smit Sibinga and his staff for putting together this very interesting and very good programme.

www.ingramcontent.com/pod-product-compliance
Ingram Content Group UK Ltd.
Pitfield, Milton Keynes, MK11 3LW, UK
UKHW021821280526
471509UK00007B/64
* 9 7 8 0 8 9 8 3 8 6 8 6 8 *